Interactions between climate and animal production

Interactions between climate and animal production

Editors:

N. Lacetera

U. Bernabucci

H.H. Khalifa

B. Ronchi

A. Nardone

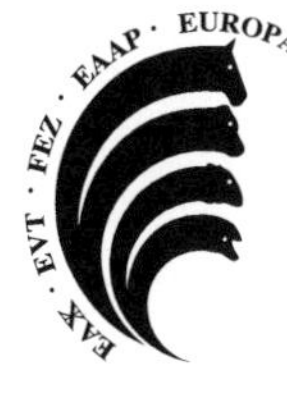

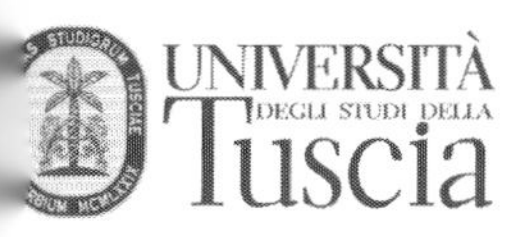

EAAP Technical Series No. 7

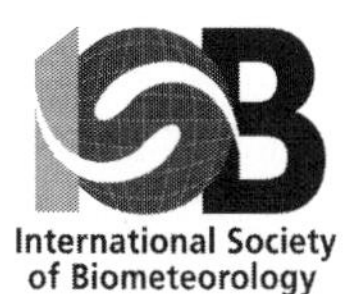

CIP-data Koninklijke Bibliotheek, Den Haag

ISBN 9076998264
ISSN 1570-7318
paperback

Subject headings:
Livestock
Hot environment
Welfare

First published, 2003

Wageningen Academic Publishers
The Netherlands, 2003

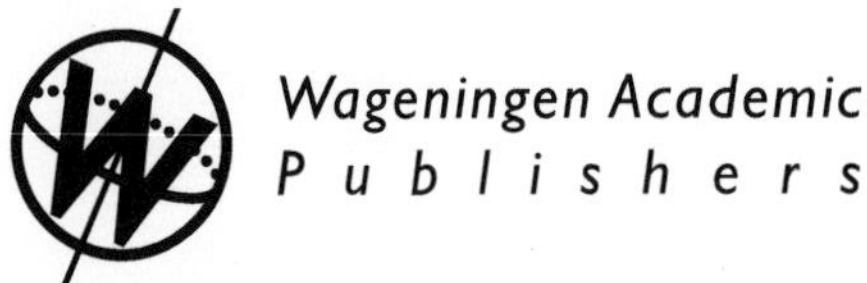

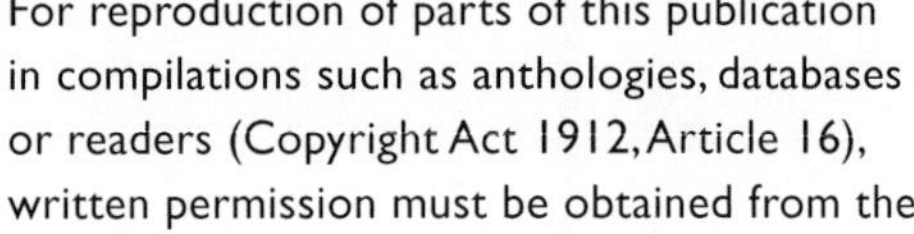

Contents

Opening remarks

A. Nardone

Dipartimento di Produzioni Animali, Via De Lellis, 01100 Viterbo, Italy, nardone@unitus.it

In the second half of last century, livestock industry has been impressively successful in its ability to improve animal performances. Such success was due to growth of scientific and technological knowledge, which permitted genetic selection of high yielding animals, adjustment of rational feeding strategies, establishment of efficacious interventions for disease prevention and therapy, and adoption of sophisticated management schemes in adapted housings.

A negative consequence of such dramatic improvement of animal performance has been a higher incidence of problems linked with metabolic vulnerability and with the reduced capacity of selected animals to adapt to stressful conditions.

Specialisation and intensification of animal production also contributed to a reduction in the number of breeds. A few genetic types selected for high performances (Friesian and Brown among milk cattle breeds, Large White and Landrace among swine, a few lines in poultry) gradually replaced a number of breeds adapted to different environments with different climates. These processes were more evident in the so called industrialised countries where temperate climate is often predominant and optimal for high yielding selected animals.

Climate is a dynamic phenomenon as demonstrated by changes of the temperature of our planet over the last 35 millions years (fluctuation occurred on a large scale periods as determined through the isotope O_{18}, as well as on shorter terms like in the last 1000 years). Nevertheless, climatic data referred to last years appear quite alarming: from 1860 the temperature of the earth is increasing gradually and the last decade has been the hottest of the last six centuries as ascertained through the analysis of trees rings and lake sediments. Recent evolution of climatic conditions was due to variation of natural phenomena (i.e. solar radiation) or was caused by the greenhouse effect linked to the increase of CO_2 (from 280 ppm to 350 ppm in a little more than two centuries), methane (from 800 to 1700 ppm) and nitrous oxide (from 285 to 310) caused above all by some human activities. The latter data testify that it is becoming quite urgent a clarification about the necessity to change human behaviour and also to modify selection, feeding and housing strategies of livestock.

Furthermore, some situations referred to large geographic area make still more urgent provision of answers and possibly identification of novel strategies:

- the increase of animal products consumption at a rate higher than animal production capabilities. This because of a rapid increase of human population and per capita consumption in several countries placed in tropical or subtropical regions;
- the difficulties to obtain high productivity from selected animals in several developing countries due to low management capacities and to hot environment;
- the extinction of several local breeds due to the spreading of intensive systems (the FAO reports that in the last century about 1000 breeds vanished and that today about further 1300 are at risk of extinction).

In order to these problems, can we consider appropriate the level of knowledge on animal adaptation and management in severe climatic conditions? Which moment of the animal husbandry still need to be reinforced to satisfy requirements of livestock reared in such unfavourable conditions? Could the selection strategies and objectives be modified to obtain animals well-adapted and productive in extreme conditions? The heritability of some anatomical or morphological traits or physiological process involved in maintaining thermal balance seems high enough to hypothesise such solution, at least for dairy cattle. The new approach of using the recent tools of biotechnology, in particular the possibility to find molecular markers associated to QTLs or genes, or that to detect directly genetic variants, could help to get to the goal in short time, in contrast to the length of a number of generations as quantitative genetic requires.

Finally, to what extent the higher number and productivity of farm animals affect climate and which are the possible solution to this emerging problem to safeguard the environmental integrity for the future generations?

I am confident this Symposium will provide useful answers to several questions and I hope it will represent the first of a series of qualified exchanges of knowledge and experiences between animal scientists and animal biometeorologists.

Bioclimatology and adaptation of farm animals in a changing climate

H.H. Khalifa

Al-Azhar University, Faculty of Agriculture, Animal production Department, 11884, Nasr City, Cairo, Egypt, e-mail: khalifahhk@usa.net

Summary

Bioclimatology plays a key role in the mitigation of climatic impacts on animal production. In arid and semi-arid regions, high ambient temperature accompanied with scarcity of water affects significantly animal production to be about 2-4% of world meat, milk and egg production. General circulation models (GCMs) of climatic changes indicate that rising levels of greenhouse gases are likely to increase the global average surface temperature by 1.5-4.5 C over the next 100 years, raise sea-levels, amplify extreme weather events such as storms and hot spells, shift climate zones poleward, and reduce soil moisture. Farm animals will be affected directly and indirectly by these climatic changes resulting in a substantial reduction in meat, milk and egg production. Study of animal adaptation mechanisms and managerial techniques to alleviate the effect of extreme climates and climatic changes on animal will help in mitigation of climatic impacts on animal production. The aim is to discuss the bioclimatic factors causing necessity of farm animal adaptation as well as adaptive mechanisms to mitigate the impacts of climate on animal performance to overcome the gap between human demands and animal production.

Keywords: biometeorology, adaptation, climatic changes, animal production

Introduction

There are massive pressures on animal production to satisfy the deeply rooted demand for high value animal protein. These pressures are resulting in a major transformation of the livestock sector, from one which is resource-driven to one that looks aggressively for new resources. Livestock are not only important as producers of meat, milk and eggs, which are part of the modern food chain and provide high value protein food, but other non-food functions still provide the rationale for keeping the majority of the world's livestock. Often, livestock constitute the main, if not the only, capital reserve of farming households, serving as a strategic reserve that reduces risk and adds stability to the overall farming system (Steinfeld, 1998). The gap between animal production and human demand is mainly due to climatic and economic factors. The impacts of climate on animal production include the effect of extreme climates as well as the effect of global climatic changes.

The sub-Saharan Africa (SSA) and West Asia and North Africa (WANA) geographical regions produce about 2-4.5% of the world animal production as meat, milk or egg. According to the Agro-ecological classification (Sere & Steinfeld, 1996), temperate and tropical highlands mixed farm rainfed (MRT) produce 38.6 of the world meat production (beef and veal) and 55.5% of the world total milk productions compared with the 4.5 of world meat and 9.3% of world total milk production produce from Arid semi-Arid tropics and subtropics (MRA). In addition, 21.3% of pig production comes from MRT, while MRA produce only 0.5% of world production. On the other hand, poultry production (meat and egg and rabbit) do not differ between geographic or climatic regions where 73.9% of world

poultry meat and 67.9% of world egg productions come from livestock landless monogastric system (LLM).
United Nations Environment Program Information Unit for Climate Change Fact Sheet 101 studied the impacts of climatic changes on agriculture (UNEP, 1990). The general circulation models (GCMs) indicate that rising levels of greenhouse gases are likely to increase the global average surface temperature by 1.5-4.5 C over the next 100 years, raise sea-levels (thus inundating farmland and making coastal groundwater saltier), amplify extreme weather events such as storms and hot spells, shift climate zones poleward, and reduce soil moisture. Higher levels of CO2 should stimulate photosynthesis in C3 plants (include such major mid-latitude food staples as wheat, rice, and soybean). The response of C4 plants, on the other hand, would not be as dramatic (C4 plants include such low-latitude crops as maize, sorghum, sugar-cane, and millet, plus many pasture and forage grasses). Because average temperatures are expected to increase more near the poles than near the equator, the shift in climate zones will be more pronounced in the higher latitudes. In the mid-latitude regions (45 to 60 latitude), the shift is expected to be about 200-300 kilometres for every degree Celsius of warming. The greatest risks for low-latitude countries are that reduced rain fall and soil moisture will damage crops in semi-arid regions, and that additional heat stress will damage crops and especially livestock in humid tropical regions. Valtorta (2002) has discussed the direct and indirect impacts of climate on animal production.
According to climatic change scenarios, milk production in hot/hot-humid southern regions of United States might decline by 5-14%, conception rate will be reduced by 36% and short-term extreme events (e.g. summer heat wave and winter storms) can result in the death of vulnerable animals (IPCC, 2001).
The impacts of global changes on livestock performance have been analyzed and discussed by Hahn et al. (2002). They reported that the percent increase in days to market for swine and beef, and the percent decrease in dairy milk production, for the 2030 scenarios averaged 1.2, 2.0, and 2.2%, respectively, using the CGCMI model, and 0.9, 0.7, and 2.1%, respectively, for the Hadley model. For the 2090 scenario, respective changes averaged 13.1, 6.9, and 6.0% for the CGCMI model and 4.3, 3.4, and 3.9% using the Hadley model.
Animal adaptation and alleviation of the detrimental effects of extreme climates on livestock production will overcome the gap between livestock production and human demands especially in arid and semiarid tropical and subtropical regions, as well as the expected effect of climatic changes on animal production in mid-latitude and temperate zones. Biometeorology plays a key role in the assessment of climatic impacts of atmospheric variation and variability upon stress, morbidity and mortality in animals and humans (including physiological and psychological adaptations) and systems for lessening those effects (ISB, 2003).

Bioclimatology, ecology, environmental physiology and biometeorology

Animal bioclimatology is the science deals with the inter-relationships between climate, soil, plants and animals (Hafez, 1968a). In 1974, Folk defined animal environmental physiology as the science deals with the study of healthy mammals in relation to their natural physical environment as studied in Geophysics. Figure 1 demonstrates the relationship between concepts of Environmental physiology, Bioclimatology, Biometeorology and Ecology (Folk, 1974).
The International Society of Biometeorology (ISB) founded on 1956 decided at first to support the term Bioclimatology then changed the name of their discipline of study to Biometeorology (Folk, 1974). ISB web site stated that Biometeorology is an interdisciplinary science studying the interactions between atmospheric processes and living organisms - plants, animals and humans. It concerns the process-response system of energy and matter

flows within the biosphere (ISB, 2003). According to ISB definition and scopes, the concept of Biometeorology as an integrative and interdisciplinary science includes Environmental physiology, Bioclimatology and Ecology.
This paper deals with the farm animal biometeorology as one of the scopes of ISB - Animal Biometeorolgy Commission and will be focused on the interaction between climate and farm animal production. The description of bioclimatic factors causing necessity of farm animal adaptation, the morphological, physiological and behavioral adaptation mechanisms of different farm animals to natural changes and to extremes of the physical environment as well as methods to mitigate the impacts of climate on animal performance (morbidity and mortality) will be discussed.

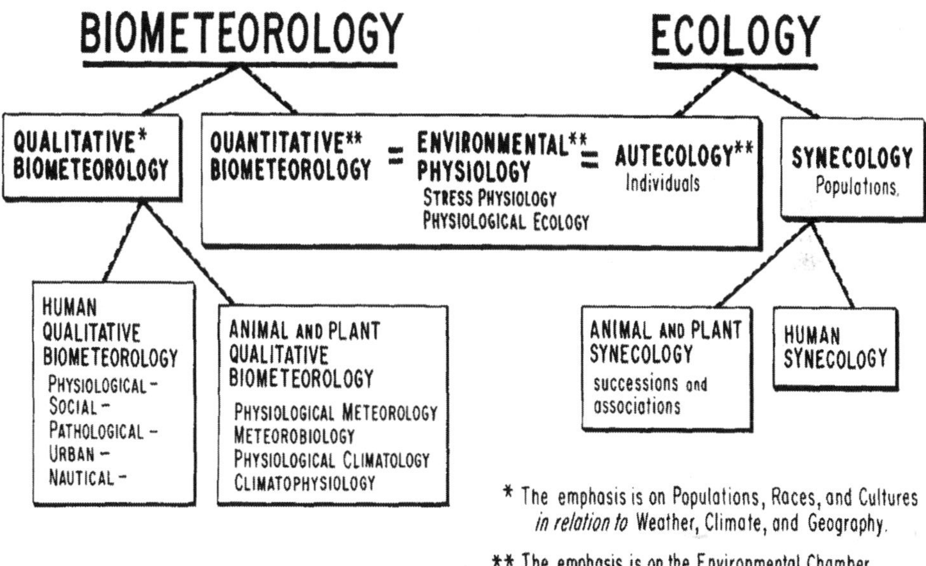

Figure 1. Relationship between Biometeorology and Ecology (Folk, 1974).

Climatic factors affecting livestock

According to Koeppen (1936) and from the biometeorology point of view, climatic regions can be classified according to its effect on animals to: hot, cold and altitude (Table 1). Folk (1974) and Hahn et al., (2003) demonstrated that the main natural physical environmental factors affecting livestock are: air temperature, relative humidity, radiant heat, precipitation, atmospheric pressure, ultraviolet light, wind velocity and dust.
Impacts of climatic factors on farm animal production, reproduction, morbidity and mortality are illustrated in Tables (2-5). It is worth noting that the effect climate on farm animals depends greatly on the severity and duration of climatic factor and animal adaptive mechanism. Chronic heat stress for example affects animal morbidity, production and reproduction, while it has a slight effect on animal mortality. Meanwhile, acute heat stress may increase mortality rate especially when drinking water is not available. Khalifa (1999) and Khalifa et al. (2000) demonstrated that it is important to study the effect of heat stress on mortality rate to evaluate the best method to alleviate the effect of heat stress on broilers. Moreover, to mitigate the effect

of climate on different farm animals, biometeorologist must study the main effect of climate on different animals as well as the adaptive and managerial mechanisms to alleviate this effect. For example, the main cause of high mortality rate in broilers under heat stress is due to a low plasma albumin concentration during summer causing an interstitial edema and low plasma and blood volumes. Consequently, the addition of electrolytes or bicarbonate will not improve mortality rate during heat stress although it may improve some physiological parameters (body temperature and respiration rate). Furthermore, early acclimation of broilers to heat stress at 1 week of age may be the best method to alleviate the effect of heat stress on mortality rate by producing heat shock proteins. He concluded that some of the managerial manipulations to mitigate the effect of heat stress on broiler chicks improved productive performance and some adaptive parameters; meanwhile, they have no role in the alleviation of mortality rate or their role need more investigations.

Table 1. Classification of climates according to their main effects on animals.

Climate	Region	Koeppen classification	Main effect
Hot			
Hot wet climate	Tropical and subtropical	A and C	Heat stress in summer, rain, wind, storm
Hot dry climate	Low latitude, arid (desert)	B	Heat stress in summer, salinity, dehydration, starvation
	High latitude, semiarid		Cold stress in winter
Cold	Savana	Aw	Cold stress in winter
	Arid and semiarid	B	Cold stress in winter
	Polar	E	Cold stress, rain
Altitude	Moist Continental Mid-latitude	D	Cold stress, low pressure

Table 2. Impact of hot climate on animal productivity.

Productive trait	Effect	Reference
Maintenance requirement	Increase	Ames (1986)
Feed intake	Decrease	Ames (1986) and Ronchi et al. (2002)
Milk production	Decrease	El-Nouty et al. (1989) and Valtorta et al. (2002)
Daily gain	Decrease	Sakaguchi and Gaughan (2002)
Egg production	Decrease	Anjum et al. (2002)
Egg shell thickness	Decrease	North and Bell (1990)
Wool production	Increase	Woods et al. (1995)

Table 3. Impact of cold climate on animal productivity.

Productive trait	Effect	Reference
Maintenance requirement	increase	Ames (1986)
Feed intake	increase	Ekpe and Christopherson (2000)
Milk production	decrease (below -5°C)	Johnson (1986b) & Leva et al. (1996)
Daily gain	Decrease (below 0°C)	Johnson (1986a)
Egg production	Decrease below 9°C	Hafez (1986b)
Egg shell thickness	No effect	
Wool production	decrease	Woods et al. (1995)

Table 4. Impact of hot climate on animal reproductive performance.

Reproductive trait	Effect	Reference
Puberty	Heat stress delay puberty in both males and females	Fuquay (1986)
	Photoperiod and the moderate high ambient temperature during summer improved sexual respond	Abdalla (1996)
Spermatogenesis and semen quality	Higher volume and quality of semen during summer	Abdalla (1996)
	High ambient temperatures (27 to 40 °C) reduced semen quality	Kelly and Hurst (1963)
Estrous cycle and ovulation	Heat stress decreases the length and intensity of estrous	Lucy (2002)
Fertilization and conception rate	Heat stress after the onset of estrous or early during the post-breeding impaired fertilization and embryonic development	Lucy (2002) & Putney et al., (1989)
Gestation	Heat stress during middle and late gestation result in smaller offspring at parturition	Ealy et al., (1993) & Fuquay (1986)
Fertility and hatchability	Fertility is affected by climate and adaptability.	
	A drop of 15-20% in hatchability whenever the mean weekly temperature exceeded 27 °C.	Jayarajan, (1992) Daghir (1995)
	Hatchability of eggs was 5 % lower during hot season than during the remainder of the year	North and Bell (1990)

Table 5. Impact of climate on animal morbidity and mortality.

Category	Effect	Reference
Non-infectious diseases	Increased	Kelley (1986)
Resistance to diseases (immunity)		
Hot or cold weather	Decreased	Kelley (1982)
Moderate heat stress (THI=72±2.6)	No effect	Lacetera (2002)
Microbial insult due to thermoregulatory behavior (huddling, seeking shade and migration)	Increased	Kelley (1986)
Disease resistance due to availability and quality of foodstuffs	Decreased	Kelley (1986) & Ronchi et al. (2002)
Mortality due to heat waves		
Broilers	Increased	Khalifa (1999)
Poultry	Increased	Etches et al. (1995)
Feedlot cattle	Increased	Hahn et al. (2000)
Dairy and beef cattle	Increased	Hahn et al. (2002)

Responses of animals to climatic changes and extreme climates

Livestock are homeothermic animals, which have the ability to control their body temperature within a narrow range under a wide range of environmental temperature. Homeostasis is the process of maintaining a constant internal environment (body temperature, body water, blood pressure, pH and ionic equilibrium) despite variation in the external environment. However, McLean (1991) demonstrated that mammals do not have precise control over core temperature. Accordingly, homeothermy is not a mammalian characteristic. The rigidity (or lability) of body temperature varies among species as response of adaptation. The ability to vary core temperature is known as heterothermy and may play a siginificant role in animal adaptation especially under desert conditions.

Heat balance

In its simplest form, thermal balance is expressed as:
Heat production (HP) = heat loss (LS) + heat gain (HG) ± heat storage (HS) (1)
The contribution mechanisms of heat production and heat loss and factors affecting them are shown in tables (6 & 7).

Table 6. Heat production mechanisms and factors affecting it.

Mechanisms of heat production	Factors affecting
Basal metabolic rate (BMR)	Feed consumption; hormonal control: T3, T4 and glucocorticoids; Ta or THI, behavior (hibernation, estivation, elementary)
Specific dynamic action of food (SDA)	Feed consumption; ration ingredients (roughage); rumen micro-organisms; behavior (selective feeding)
Muscle activity (MA)	
Shivering	Involuntary (hypothalamic control through skin receptors)
Exercise	Voluntary, behavior (increase locomotive activity)

Basal metabolism reflects the energy requirement for a given animal in the fasting and resting state.

Table 7. Heat loss mechanisms and factors affecting it.

Mechanisms of heat loss	Advantages	Disadvantages	Factors affecting
Physical	Water conservation (water balance)	Blocked when Ta=Tb heat gain if Ta>Tb	Temperature gradient; solar radiation & behavior
Conduction			Thermal conductivity
Internal (Cd)			Blood volume*; peripheral circulation
External (Cd)			Temperature gradient; insulation (S.B. fat, coat)
Convection (Co)	High under desert and pasture conditions		Wind velocity
Radiation (R)			Temperature gradient; solar radiation and clouds
Evaporation (E)	The only way if Ta≥Tb	Affects water balance	Air saturation (RH%); water availability
Skin	Do not affect blood pH	Blocked at high RH% Affects plasma osmolality**	
Respiratory	May cause blood alkalosis	Do not affect plasma Osmolality continued at high RH%	

Ta = Ambient temperature; Tb = Body temperature; S.B. = Subcutaneous; Internal Cd = Internal conduction from core to surface; External Cd = External conduction from surface to environment; *Factors affecting blood volume includes: ADH, Aldosterone, plsama osmolality, plasma Na^+, K^+ and albumin concentrations; **Decrease plasma osmolality due to the decrease in plasma Na^+ or K^+ concentration

Substituting mechanisms of heat production and heat loss in equation (1)

$$BMR + SDA + MA = E \pm Cd \pm Co \pm R \pm HS \pm HG \quad (2)$$

Temperature gradient is the main factor affecting this equation. If ambient temperature equal or greater than body surface temperature, animal will gain heat by Cd, Co and R and heat balance will be disturbed

$$HP + Cd + Co + R > E + HS \quad (3)$$

Regulation of body temperature

The temperature regulating system consists of three basic components (Figure 2-a & b): sensors (peripheral cold and warm receptors), a thermostatic control unit consists of heat loss center (anterior hypothalamus) and heat production center (posterior hypothalamus) thermoregulatory effectors (peripheral vasoconstriction or dilatation, sweating, panting, shivering and non-shivering or endocrine). The thermostatic control unit seeks to maintain the core body temperature (central body temperature) close to a set-point and the control of effectors (heat loss and heat production) is based on the difference between the actual core temperature and the desired core temperature (Bianca, 1968). Bligh (1966) has discussed the variable set-point hypothesis for thermoregulatory effectors responses to the difference between actual and required hypothalamic temperatures.

Physical and/or physiological mechanisms are the most important thermoregulatory adjustments of farm animals to thermoneutral environment. The physiological mechanisms involve muscular, cardiovascular and metabolic changes, while physical mechanisms involve involuntary activation of somatic reflexes and voluntary behavioral adjustments (Macfarlane, 1964). The behavioral adjustments include postural changes, changes in food intake and water consumption, diurnal and nocturnal patterns in activity, hibernation, locomotors activities and shelter or shade seeking.

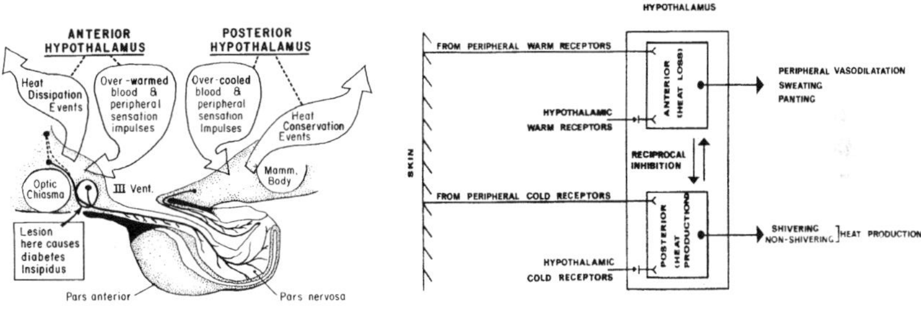

Figure 2. a: Probable physiological processes associated with control of temperature regulation by hypothalamic structures (Folk, 1974). b: Simplified representation of the temperature regulating system (Bianca, 1968, adapted from Bligh, 1964/1965, Vet. Annual, 246).

Limits of thermoregulation in heat and cold

The zone of survival and its classification to zones of hypothermy, homeothery and hyperthermy is illustrated in Figure 3. The temperature limits of survival zone (D – D'), zone of homeothermy (C – C'), zone of thermoneutrality (B – B') and zone of thermal comfort (A –

A') are depend on changes in core body temperature and metabolic rate. Within the zone of homeothermy, animal can maintain a constant or steady state core temperature.

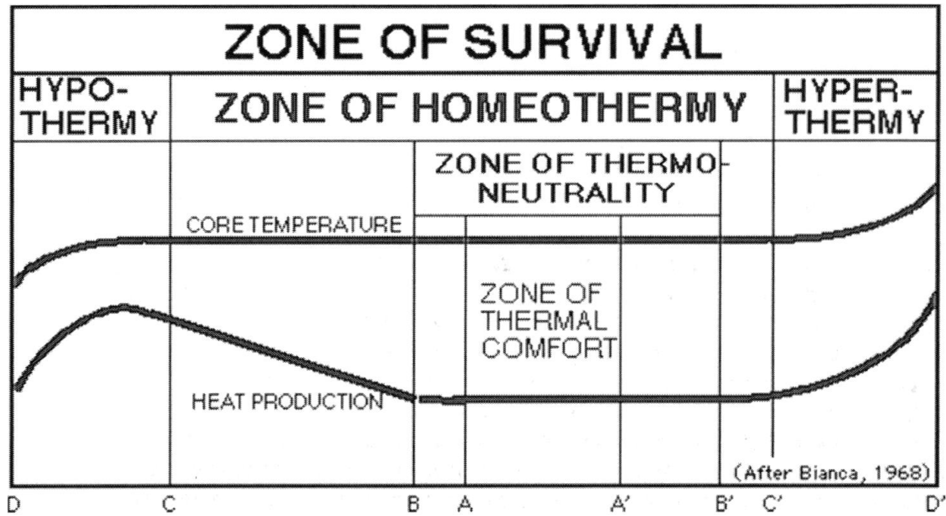

Figure 3. Zone of survival (Bianca, 1968).

Thermoneutral zone and critical environmental temperatures

The thermoneutral zone is characterized by the minimum heat production with steady state core temperature. Within the zone of thermal comfort, there is little sensation of heat or cold, and steady state core temperature can be maintained without any need for physiological or behavioral adaptation (expanding or contracting the blood vessels of the skin, evaporating excessive moisture, fluffing fur, or responding behaviorally).
At the lower critical temperature (B), heat production increases (by shivering and non-shivering thermogenesis) to maintain homeothermy. However, at the upper critical temperature (B'), increased sweating and (or) panting may be associated with lowered metabolic heat production at C', further intensification of sweating and (or) panting cannot maintain homeothermy, and the animal becomes hyperthermic. The rise in core temperature increases the metabolic rate via the van't Hoff effect (two-to three-fold rise in heat production caused by an 10°C rise in tissue temperature, Q_{10}=2-3), triggering positive feedback, which further increases the core temperature.

Critical temperatures and thermal indices

Hahn et al. (2003) discussed and compared different thermal indices for animals. They stated that the principal physical factors involved in the heat exchange process are air temperature and moisture content, thermal radiation, and airflow. Although air temperature is generally the principal driving force for heat exchange, it has long been recognized that temperature alone is rarely an adequate expression of the impact of the environment on living organisms, as it does not fully recognize the modifying influence of the other physical factors. For cold-weather conditions, Ames and Insley (1974) developed wind-chill equations for cattle and sheep, which recognize the considerable effect of hair coat on heat exchange with the surroundings. At the present time, the THI has become a standard for classifying thermal environments in many animal studies and selection of management practices during seasons other than winter.

Concept of a new animal response threshold

Based on the conclusions of Hahn et al. (2003) the use of THI instead of Ta to determine the upper critical temperature of different farm animals will correct the error of humidity effect especially under hot wet climate. Parkhurst et al. (2002) discussed the importance of stress duration in definition of heat stress threshold in bases of the transition threshold (upper critical temperature), challenge threshold and recovery (decline in body temperature after climbing). Hahn et al. (2003) discussed the importance of stress duration, intensity and recovery in THI calculation as well as the THI-hrs and recovery hours importance. The Livestock Weather Safety Index (LWSI; LCI, 1970) describes categories of heat stress associated with hot-weather conditions. The concept of the new upper critical temperature depends on the relation between THI with heat production, core temperature and evaporative cooling (respiration rate fro simplicity). The moderate heat stress will be the THI after which the respiration rate increases without any increase in core temperature or heat production. The severe heat stress (danger) is the THI after which the three physiological parameters start to increase. The correlation between these parameters (upper limit of the comfort zone and upper limit of the thermoneutral zone) with productive traits e.g. milk yield, daily gain, egg production and mortality rate due to heat stress may give a good index to predict the effect of climate on animal production and survivability. Moreover, the use of black globe temperature instead of dry bulb temperature in THI calculation (the Heat Load Index as suggested by Gaughan et al., 2002) must be considered.

Animal responses to different climates (animal adaptation)

Adaptation science describes the study of the adjustments that are possible in practices, processes or structure of systems in order to adjust to changes. The atmospheric changes causing necessity of adaptation can include: shifts in climate, declines in air quality or changes in UV levels but the term adaptation has been more commonly associated with the climate change issue (Auld et al., 2002). The concept of animal adaptation refers to the genetic and physiological changes taking place in an animal in response to internal and external stimuli. Genetic adaptation concerns selection by nature and man, whereas physiological adaptation concerns changes occurring within an individual, over shorter or longer periods. Other related concepts are acclimatization, acclimation, habituation, learning and conditioning.

Genetic and biochemical adaptation

Storey (1998) stated that in mammalian systems, ERKs are primarily responsive to growth factors and mitogens, hypoxia or osmotic stresses (Seko et al., 1996; Matsuda et al., 1995). JNKs respond to UV irradiation, heat shock, and protein synthesis inhibitors (Kyriakis et al., 1994). The third MAPK is activated by various environmental stresses (Han et al., 1994; Raingeaud et al., 1995). Storey (2001) stated that Thousands of examples of protein adaptation are known that create variants with features tailored to multiple needs including cell-, organ- or species-specific jobs, as well as to deal the effects of environmental parameters including temperature, salinity, pH, and pressure to name a few. Specific synthesis

of selected key proteins is clearly a part of animal response to environmental stress both for stress-intolerant species e.g. heat-shock proteins and stress-tolerant organisms.
Khalifa (1999) concluded that heat acclimation at early age is the best method to alleviate the effect of acute and chronic heat stress on broilers may be due to heat-shock protein (HSP) that involved in the assembly of proteins or protein containing complexes during early life of broilers (Daghir, 1995). This field of study need more investigations to know the role of genetic and biochemical adaptations in the mitigation of heat stress.

Morphological adaptations

The main morphological adaptations of different farm animals are external insulation (coat and fur thickness and subcutaneous fat), fat storage in hump or tail especially under desert conditions, skin color and body size. The most important morphological adaptation is the body size, which affects both heat production and heat loss (Grauvogl, 1996). With increasing body size the surface/volume ratio of the body increase which decrease the relative surface area and heat loss. Heat acclimated animals are more thin than cold acclimated ones to increase heat loss by increasing surface area. It is worth noting that coat insulation may be of a significant role under direct solar radiation where unshorn sheep can tolerate heat stress and water deprivation more than shorn ones (Khalifa, 1982 and Khalifa et al., 1991).
Tables (8, 9 & 10) illustrate the physiological, behavioral and morphological adaptations to different climates.

Table 8. Physiological responses to heat and cold.

Heat	Cold
Decreasing heat production Decreasing BMR or heat production Decreasing thyroid activity	Increase heat production Shivering (first defense) Exercise Imperceptible tensing of muscles Chemical increase of metabolic rate (increase glucocorticoids and thyroid hormones) Specific dynamic action of food (increase feed intake)
Increasing heat loss Increase skin evaporation (sweating) Increase respiratory evaporation (panting) Increasing internal conduction (skin circulation or vasodilatation) Increase external insulation (shorter fur or coat) Increasing insensible water loss Increasing radiating surface Increasing air movement (convection)	Decreasing heat loss Decreasing evaporative cooling through sweating and/or panting Decreasing internal conduction (vasoconstriction) Decreasing tissue conductance Increasing external insulation (length and density of fur or coat) Counter-current heat exchange
Increase heat storage which: decreases heat gain (decrease temperature gradient) and water loss through evaporation (water conservation mechanism)	

Table 9. Behavioral responses for heat and cold (Hafez, 1968c).

Heat		Cold	
Mammals	Birds	Mammals	Birds
Wallowing & rooting	Extension of wings	Hibernation	Fluffed feathers
Licking body surfaces	Feet off soil		Head under wing
Night grazing	Throwing water on comb		Covering of feet & legs
succulent feeds	Water splashing		Torpidity
	Moistening incubated eggs		Incubation & broodiness
anorexia		body flexure	
body extension		huddling	
group dispersion		extra locomotor activities	
excessive drinking		nest building	
decreased locomotor activities		seeking microclimates with higher	
moistening body surface	temperature		
seeking lower temperature			

Table 10. Main morphological adaptations in farm animals (after Hafez, 1968d).

Environmental stress	Morphological adaptation	Animal
Solar radiation	Long limbs	Camel
	Long open coat	Desert sheep and goats
High temperature	Hair shedding in summer	Camel and sheep
	Increased surface area (skin folds)	Brahman cattle
	Small body long ears	rabbit
	Loose, coarse wool	Awassi sheep
	Fine, dense wool	Merino sheep
Low temperature	Long and fine hair	Temperate cattle
	Thick subcutaneous fat	Arctic species
	Abundant brown fat	Different species
	Thick, heavy coat	Rabbit, sheep
High humidity	Dark pigmentation, sparsely haired	buffalo
Seasonality in food	Adipose tissue reserves	Awassi sheep
	Hump	camel
	Fat-tail	sheep
	Fat-rump	sheep (Somalia)
Desert	thick skin, hard tissue around mouth;	Camel
	thick mouth, lined with long papillae	
	increased drinking capacity,	
	hump (for pseudo-water storage)	
	conservation of metabolic water	
	ability to survive dehydration	
High altitude	increased O2 carrying power in blood	llama, alpaca
	increased concentration of RBCs	
	ability to transfer O2 from capillary	
	blood to tissue cells	
	high efficiency in nutrients extraction	

Comparative animal adaptations to extreme environments

Under desert conditions, the main climate impacts are high temperature and scarcity of water. Camel tolerate these impacts mainly by physiological adaptation (increasing heat storage, decreasing sensible water loss, maintaining plasma volume, special nucleated red blood cells tolerate high osmotic pressure, low metabolic rate and water turnover rate. The main behavioral mechanisms are posture, while the main morphological adaptations are foot pad, fat storage in hump, coat shedding in summer and mouth anatomy (Table, 8). On the other hand, the desert rabbit depends more on behavioral adaptation than in physiological adaptation. The nocturnal habits enables it to live in tunnels during day time with 5°C temperature than the environment and produce enough metabolic water to cover most of its requirement. Sheep and goats are less heat tolerant than camel, however, they are more adapted to desert climate than other livestock. Khalifa et al. (2002) compared adaptable response of sheep and goats to exposure to direct solar radiation and concluded that native Egyptian sheep are more tolerant to heat stress under direct solar radiation than goats may be because of their coat insulative properties.

Under cold stress, the first animal response is shivering thermogenesis to increase heat production until glucocorticoids and thyroid hormones (T3 and T4) increased through the direct effect of cold stress on hypothalamus (El-Nouty et al., 1989).

Conclusions

As an interdisciplinary science studying the interactions between atmospheric processes and living organisms - plants, animals and humans, Biometeorology concerns the process-response system or adaptive mechanisms of animals to climatic changes. The main impacts of climatic changes and extreme events can be summarized in the effect of hot, cold and high altitude. The duration, intensity and recovery of any climatic stress are the most important factors affecting farm animal production, reproduction, morbidity and mortality. The wide definition of animal adaptation is how an animal can survive and produce under the specific climate. Many physiological parameters have been used as an indication of animal adaptability to different climates i.e. body temperature and respiration rate. Researches should be aware that using these parameters alone is rarely an adequate expression of the impact of the environment on living organisms, as it does not fully recognize the modifying influence of the other physical factors. The lethal temperatures for example is very important to determine survivability of different animals to climatic changes. Climatic impacts on production and reproduction are good indicators for animal adaptability. Consequently, correlations between physiological parameters, productive and reproductive parameters and climatic changes will lead to an adequate index of animal adaptability. The following considerations are important in biometeorological studies to evaluate the adaptability of farm animals to climatic changes:

- acclimation to heat stress at early ages may be one of the most effective methods to decrease mortality under heat stress, may be through the production of heat shock proteins;
- genetic adaptation and heat shock proteins play an important role as adaptive mechanisms against climatic stress or changes. More investigations are necessary to evaluate the role of heat shock proteins and its relation to heat acclimation as an easy and economic applicable managerial manipulation against heat waves;
- biometeorologists have to take in consideration the different effects of climatic stressors on morbidity and mortality in addition to physiological, reproductive and productive responses;
- a new thermal index was suggested taking in consideration the relation between THI, metabolic rate, core temperature and respiration rate to determine the upper critical THI for

the comfort and thermoneutral zones. The use of black globe temperature instead of dry bulb temperature in the calculation of THI (the Heat Load Index) has to be evaluated. The severity of stress can be evaluated according to changes in productivity and mortality in relation to changes in body temperature, respiration rate, metabolic rate and black global temperature. Duration and severity of THI must be evaluated;
- to study the main morphological, behavioral and physiological adaptive mechanisms against climatic changes in different farm animals under different physiological status.

References

Abdalla E.B., 1996. Effect of season and surgical deviation of penis on semen characteristics and peripheral testosterone concentration in a Awassi rams. In: Proc. 9th Conf. Egypt. Soc. Anim. Prod. 371-378.

Ames D.R., 1986. Assessing the impact climate. Limiting the effects of stress on cattle. In: Moberg G.P. (editor), Utah Agric. Exp. St. Res. Bull. 512, Utah State University, Logan, Utah, USA, 1-6.

Ames D.A. & Insley L.W., 1974. Wind-chill effect for cattle and sheep. J. Anim. Sci. 40: 161-165.

Anjum M.S.Z. Rahman M., Akram S.M. & Sandhu M.A., 2002. Haematochemical profile of commercial layers influenced by heat combating systems during high ambient temperature. In: Proc. 15th Conf. Biometeorol. Aerobiol. 102-103.

Auld H., Maclver D., Urquizo N. & Fenech A., 2002. Biometeorology and adaptation guidelines for country studies. In: Proc. 15th Conf. Biometeorol. Aerobiol. 139-142.

Bianca W., 1968. Thermoregulation. In: Hafez E.S.E. (editor), Adaptation of domestic animals, Lea & Febiger, Philadelphia, USA, 97-118.

Bligh J., 1966. The Thermosensitivity of the Hypothalamus and Thermoregulation in Mammals. Biol. Rev. 41: 317-367.

Daghir N.J., 1995. Poultry Production in Hot Climate. CAB International, Wallingford, Oxcon OX10 8DE, UK.

Ealy R.J., McBride B.W., Vatnick L. & Bell W., 1993. Chronic heat stress and prenatal development in sheep: II Placental cellularity and metabolism. J. Anim. Sci. 69: 3610-3616.

Ekpe E.D. & Christopherson R.J., 2000. Metabolic and endocrine responses to cold and feed restriction in ruminants. Can. J. Anim. Sci. 80: 87-95.

El-Nouty F.D., Johnson H.D., Kamal T.H., Hassan G.A. & Salem M.H., 1989. Some hormonal characteristics of high and low yielding Holstein cows and water buffaloes located in temperate and subtropical environments. J. Tropic. Agric. Vet. Sci. 27: 461-468.

Etches R.J., John T.M. & Gibbins A.M.V., 1995. Behavioural, physiological, neuroendocrine and molecular responses to heat stress. In: Poultry production in hot climate. CAB International, Wallingford, Oxcon OX10 8DE, UK, pp 31-53.

Fuquay J.W., 1986. Effects of environmental stressors on reproduction. Limiting the effects of stress on cattle. In: Moberg G.P. (editor), Utah Agric. Exp. St. Res. Bull. 512, Utah State University, Logan, Utah, USA, 21-26.

Folk J.E. Jr., 1974. What is environmental physiology: history and terminology. In: textbook of environmental physiology, Lea & Febiger, Philadelphia, USA, 1-16.

Gaughan J.G., Goopy J. & Spark. J., 2002. Excessive heat load index for feedlot cattle. Meat and Livestock-Australia Project Rept, FLOT.316. MLA, Ltd., Locked Bag 991, N. Sydney NSW, 2059 Australia.

Grauvogl, A., 1996. Climate and livestock behaviour. In: Proc. 14th Int. Congr. Biometeorol. 395-401.

Hafez E.S.E., 1968a. Principles of animal adaptation. In: Hafez E.S.E. (editor), Adaptation of domestic animals, Lea & Febiger, Philadelphia, USA, 3-17.

Hafez E.S.E., 1968b. Environmental effects on animal productivity. In: Hafez E.S.E. (editor), Adaptation of domestic animals, Lea & Febiger, Philadelphia, USA, 74-96.

Hafez E.S.E., 1968c. Behavioral Adaptation. In: Hafez E.S.E. (editor), Adaptation of domestic animals, Lea & Febiger, Philadelphia, USA, 202-214.

Hafez E.S.E., 1968d. Morphological And Anatomical Adaptations. In: Hafez E.S.E. (editor), Adaptation of domestic animals, Lea & Febiger, Philadelphia, USA, 61-73.

Hahn G.L., Mader T.L. & Eigenberg R.A., 2003. Perspectives on Development of Thermal Indices for Animal Studies and Management. In: Proc. Symp. Interactions between climate and animal production. EAAP Technical Series no. 7: in press.

Hahn, G.L., Mader T.L., Gaughan J.B., Hu Q. & Nienaber J.A., 2000. Heat waves and their impacts on feedlot cattle. In Proc. 15th Int. Congr. Biometeorol. 353-357.

Hahn G.L., Mader T.L., Harrington J.A., Nienaber J.A. & Frank K.L., 2002. Living with climatic variability and potential global change: Climatological analysis of impacts on livestock performance. In: Proc. 15th Conf. Biometeorol. Aerobiol. 45-49.

Han J., Lee J-D., Bibbs L. & Ulevitch R.J.. 1994. A MAP kinase targeted by endotoxin and hyperosmolarity in mammalian cells. Science 265: 808-811.

Jayarajan, S., 1992. Seasonal variation in fertility and hatchability of chicken eggs. Ind. J. Poult. Sci. 27: 36-39.

ISB, International Society of Biometeorology, 2003. http://www.es.mq.edu.au/ISB/.

Johnson, D.E., 1986a. Climatic stress and production efficiency. Limiting the effects of stress on cattle. In: Moberg G.P. (editor), Utah Agric. Exp. St. Res. Bull. 512, Utah State University, Logan, Utah, USA, 17-20.

Johnson, H.D., 1986b. The effects of temperature and thermal balance on milk production. Limiting the effects of stress on cattle, In: Moberg G.P. (editor), Utah Agric. Exp. St. Res. Bull. 512, Utah State University, Logan, Utah, USA, 33-46

IPCC, 2001. Ecosystems and their goods and services. In: Climate change 2001. Impacts, adaptation and vulnerability. UNEP/WMO 257.

Kelly J.W. & Hurst V., 1963. The effect of season on fertility of the dairy bull and the dairy cow. J. Am. Vet. Med. Ass. 143: 40.

Kelley K.W., 1982. Immunobiology of domestic animals as affected by hot and cold weather. In. Proc. 2nd International Livestock Environment Symposium. ASAE Publ. 3–82. ASAE, St. Joseph, Mich. 470–483

Kelley K.W., 1986. Weather and animal health. Limiting the effects of stress on cattle. In: Moberg G.P. (editor), Utah Agric. Exp. St. Res. Bull. 512, Utah State University, Logan, Utah, USA, 11-16.

Khalifa H.H., 1982. Wool coat and thermoregulation in sheep under Egyptian conditions. Ph.D. Thesis, Fac. Agric., Al-Azhar, Univ., Cairo, Egypt.

Khalifa H.H., 1999. Evaluation of some managerial manipulation to alleviate the effect of heat stress on broiler chickens. In: Proc. 15th Int. Congr. Biometeorol. 117.

Khalifa H.H., El-Sherbiny A.A. & Abdel-Khalek T.M., 2002. Effect of exposure to solar radiation on thermoregulation of sheep and goats. In: Proc. 15th Conf. Biometeorol. Aerobiol. 428-432.

Khalifa H.H., Ahmad N.A., El-Tantawy S.M.T., Kicka M.A. & Dawoud A.M., 2000. Effect of heat acclimation on body fluids and plasma proteins of broilers exposed to acute heat stress. In: Proc. 11th Conf. Egypt. Soc. Anim. Prod.

Khalifa H.H., Khalil M.H. & Abdel-Bary H.T., 1991. Significance of wool coat length on physiological responses to dehydration of Barki sheep. Al-Azhar J. Agric. Res. 14: 43-48.

Koeppen G., 1936. Handbuch der Klimatologie, Verlagsbuchhandlung, Berlin.

Kyriakis J.M., Banerjee P., Nikolakaki E., Dai T., Rubie E.A., Ahmad M.F., Avruch J. & Woodgett J.R., (1994). The stress-activated protein kinase subfamily of c-jun kinases. Nature 369: 156-160.

Lacetera N., Bernabucci U., Ronchi B., Scalia D. & Nardone A., 2002. Moderate summer heat stress does not modify immunological parameters of Holstein dairy cows. Int. J. Biometeorol. 46: 33-37.

LCI, 1970. Patterns of transit losses. Livestock Conservation, Inc., Omaha, NE.

Leva P.E., Valtorta S.E. & Fornasero L.V., 1996. Milk production decline during summer in Argentina: Present situation and expected effects of global warming. In: Proc. 14th Intern. Congr. Biometeorol. 395-401.

Lucy M.C., 2002. Reproductive loss in farm animal during heat stress. In: Proc. 15th Conf. Biometeorol. Aerobiol. 50-53.

Macfarlane W.V., 1964. Terrestrial animals in dry heat. In: Dill D.B., Adolph E.F. & Wilber C.G. (editors), Adaptation to the environment, handbook of physiology, Vol. IV, Am. Physiol. Soc.Washington D.C., USA.

McLean M., 1991. A climate change mammalian population collapse mechanism. In: Kainlauri E., Johansson A., Kurki-Suonio I. & Geshwiler M. (editors), Energy and environment, ASHRAE, Atlanta, Georgia, USA, 93-100.

Matsuda S., Kawasaki H., Moriguchi T., Gotoh Y. & Nishida E. 1995. Activation of protein kinase cascades by osmotic shock. J. Biol. Chem. 270: 12781-12786.

North M.D. & Bell D., 1990. Commercial chicken production manual. 4th ed. Van Nostrand Reinhold, New York, USA, 643.

Parkhurst A.M., Spiers D.A., Mader T.L. & Hahn G.L., 2002. What is the definition of heat stress threshold. In: Proc. 15th Conf. Biometeorol. Aerobiol. 162-165.

Putney D.J., Mullins S., Thatcher W.W., Drost M. & Gross T.S., 1989. Embryonic development in superovulated dairy cattle exposed to elevated ambient temperature between the onset of estrus and insemination. Anim. Reprod. Sci. 19: 37-51.

Raingeaud J., Gupta S., Rogers J.S., Dickens M., Han J., Ulevitch R.J. & Davis R.J. 1995. Pro-inflammatory cytokines and environmental stress cause p38 mitogen-activated protein kinase activation by dual phosphorylation on tyrosine and threonine. J. Biol. Chem. 270: 7420-7426.

Ronchi B., Bernabucci U., Lacetera N. & Nardone A., 2002. Influence of different term of exposure to hot environment on diet digestibility by sheep. In: Proc. 53rd Annual Meeting EAAP 117.

Sakaguchi Y. & Gaughan J.B., 2002. The effect of heat stress on carcass characteristics of beef cattle. Reproductive loss in farm animal during heat stress. In: Proc. 15th Conf. Biometeorol. Aerobiol. 114-115.

Seko Y., Tobe K., Ueki K., Kadowaki T., & Yazaki Y., 1996. Hypoxia and hypoxia/ reoxygenation activate Raf-1, mitogen-activated protein kinase kinase, mitogen-activated protein kinases, and S6 kinase in cultured rat cardiac myocytes. Circ. Res. 78: 82-90.

Sere C. & Steinfeld H., 1996. World livestock production systems: current status, issue and trends. Animal Production and Health, paper No. 127, FAO, Rome.

Steinfeld H., 1998. Livestock and the environment. In: Proc. Intern. Conf. Livest. Env.

Storey K.B., 1998. Survival under stress: Molecular mechanisms of metabolic rate depression in animals. South African J. Zool. 33: 55.64.

Storey K.B., 2001. Turning down the fires of life: metabolic regulation of hibernation and estivation. In: Storey K.B. (editor), Molecular mechanisms of metabolic arrest, BIOS Scientific Publishers, Oxford, UK, 1-21.

Valtorta S.E., 2002. Animal production in a changing climate: Impacts and mitigation. In: Proc. 15th Conf. Biometeorol. Aerobiol. 98-101.

Valtorta S.E., Leva P.E., Gallardo M.G., & Scarpati O.S., 2002. Milk production responses during heat waves events in Argentina. In: Proc. 15th Conf. Biometeorol. Aerobiol. 98-101.

Woods J.L. Bray A.R., Rogers G.R. & Smith M.C., 1995. Seasonal patterns of wool growth in Romney sheep selected for high and low staple tenacity. In: Proc. New Zealand Soc. Anim. Prod. 55: 42-45.

UNEP, United Nations Environment Programme. 1990. The impacts of climate change on agriculture. Fact Sheet 101. UNEP Information unit for climate change (IUCC).

Perspective on development of thermal indices for animal studies and management

G.L. Hahn[1], T.L. Mader[2] & R.A. Eigenberg[1]

[1] *U.S. Meat Animal Research Center, PO Box 166, Clay Center, NE, hahn@email.marc.usda.gov, eigenberg@email.marc.usda.gov*
[2] *Extension and Research, University of Nebraska, Concord, NE, tmader@unlnotes02.unl.edu*

Summary

Heat exchanges with the environment are a crucial process for maintaining homeothermy by humans and other animals. These exchanges involve heat production, conservation and dissipation, and are dependent on both biological and physical factors. The complexity of these exchanges have led to many attempts to represent the environmental aspects by surrogate thermal indices as a basis for assessing the biological effect and consequent impact of the thermal environment. Resultant index values represent effects produced by the heat exchange process. For humans, comfort assessment is primary; for animals, assessing performance, health and well-being have been foremost. This dichotomy of approaches is discussed from the perspectives of past and current indices, and considerations for future efforts. Emphasis is on thermal indices useful in animal studies and applications, with a view toward strategic and tactical decisions for rational environmental management. Numerous illustrative examples are included.

Keywords: thermal indices, farm animals, biological response functions, research, environmental management

Introduction

Thermal climate influences living organisms through heat exchanges between the organism and its environment. Those exchanges are dependent on both biological and physical factors, and there have been many efforts to model the interactions. In the case of animals, biological factors are primarily related to heat dissipation or conservation, and include physiological and behavioral components. Thermoregulatory mechanisms are complex; for domestic animals, the relative importance of the various mechanisms varies by species. Adaptive aspects, both short- and long-term, can also be quite important elements.

Principal physical factors involved in the heat exchange process are air temperature and moisture content, thermal radiation, and airflow. Although air temperature is generally the primary driving force for heat exchange, it has long been recognized that temperature alone is rarely an adequate expression of the impact of the environment on living organisms, as it doesn't fully recognize the modifying influence of the other physical factors.

The focus of this treatise is on indices that represent the influence of thermal environments on animal responses, with particular reference to domestic livestock. Comparisons are made between indices used for human and animal applications, and between some approaches used to quantify the impact of the thermal environment on animals. Philosophical aspects are emphasized. While we do not attempt an exhaustive review of all such efforts that have been made, numerous examples are included to enhance understanding of the background and application of specific approaches used in environmental management of livestock. Finally, we suggest considerations that may be useful in the further development of thermal indices for animal studies and management applications.

General background

Temperature provides a measure of the sensible heat content of air, and represents a major portion of the driving force for sensible heat exchange between the environment and an animal. However, latent heat content of the air, as represented by some measure of the insensible heat content (e.g., dewpoint temperature), thermal radiation (short- and long-wave) and airflow also impact the total heat exchange. Because of the limitations of air temperature alone as a measure of the thermal environment, there have been many efforts to combine the effects of two or more thermal measures representing the influence of sensible and latent heat exchanges between the organism and its environment. It is important to recognize that all such efforts produce *index values*, rather than a true temperature (even when expressed on a temperature scale). As such, an index value represents the *effect* produced by the heat exchange process, which can alter the biological response that might be associated with changes in temperature alone. In the case of humans, the useful effect is the sensation of comfort; for animals, the useful effect is the impact on performance, health, and well-being.
It should also be recognized that indices are mathematical models, which never truly represent the complexity of the physical/biological interactions; for example, index relationships are typically linear, while real world relationships are not. Nevertheless, thermal indices have value, serving as surrogates for the complex interactions between the physical and biological components. Thresholds, above or below which better representation is obtained of the effect of the thermal environment, are crucial elements for consideration in the development and use of thermal indices. Further, static responses of organisms to thermal environments are generally assumed; in reality, the responses are temporally dynamic and involve interactions within the biological system.

Indices for humans

Historically, most efforts to develop thermal indices have been for human applications, with emphasis on assessment of comfort, involving both psychological and physiological aspects. Jendritzky et al. (2002) states that more than 100 such indices have been developed over the past 150 years, most of them based on two thermal parameters, to represent the complex heat exchanges between the human body and the thermal environment. Ideally,"...each index value will always result in a unique thermophysiological effect, regardless of the combination of the input meteorological input values" (Jendritzky et al., 2002). This utopian goal is unattainable in reality because of personal factors (e.g., clothing, training, acclimatization) and the complexity of the environment. Table 29.4 of the Handbook of Applied Meteorology (edited by Houghton, 1985) lists representative biometeorological indices developed for human applications, ranging from the simple to the complex.
For evaluation of human environments, Houghten & Yaglou (1923) reported on an "effective temperature" (ET), which combined the effects of air temperature and humidity with wind speed (no thermal radiation load). The ET was then related to the perceived comfort of human test subjects in an environmental chamber. Results, applicable for moderate to hot conditions, were presented as a nomogram, with percentages of comfortable subjects at various conditions. These research results have subsequently been used in the selection of design criteria for heating and air-conditioning systems for human housing.
For cold conditions, Siple & Passel (1945) developed a wind-chill index (WCI), relating air temperature and windspeed to the time for freezing of a small cylinder of water, which served as a rough guide for protecting against frostbite of human skin exposed to cold conditions. Because of the lack of recognition of the biological element of the response to cold in the WCI, there have been various attempts to improve that index in recent years. An Internet

"Wind-Chill Workshop," hosted by Environment Canada, was held in early 2000 <http:/windchill.ec.gc.ca./workshop/sessions/index_e.html>, and Environment Canada has also reported on a new wind-chill equation based on heat transfer from the human face to its surroundings. This equation, now in use in both Canada and the United States, can be accessed at the website: <www.msc.ec.gc.ca/education/windchill/science_equations_e.cfm>, (created in August, 2002 and modified January, 2003).

A "Discomfort Index" (DI) was proposed by Earl Thom of the U.S. Weather Bureau (Thom, 1959) to classify levels of discomfort for humans during the summer months, based on air drybulb temperature (TDB) and humidity (RH) or other measure of air moisture content (wetbulb, TWB; dewpoint, TDP). The DI could then be used with climatological records to evaluate likelihood of occurrences of discomfort levels at various locations. However, some locations portrayed as being highly likely to have uncomfortable weather conditions were tourist attractions, so the DI was renamed the Temperature-Humidity Index (THI)[1]. Hendrick (1959) also suggested an outdoor Weather Comfort Index which included air temperature, humidity, windspeed, and solar radiation components, but it failed to gain general usage.

Currently, the U.S. National Weather Service uses the comfort-based Heat Index (HI) for forecasts during hot conditions. Watts & Kalkstein (2002) have proposed a Heat Stress Index (HSI) based on the HI, but modified to reflect cloud cover, cooling degree-days, consecutive day count of elevated HI, and adaptive aspects of people in different locales. While based on human comfort, the HSI has also been correlated with human mortality in areas with thermal extremes, such as heat waves (Watts & Kalkstein, 2002). This provides a measure of associated risk that can be used in forecasts.

It is recognized that these relatively simple indices for moderate to hot conditions have limitations, and there have been many efforts to improve on them. Quite recently, several biometeorologists from around the world have been collaborating to develop an index with universal relevance for human applications based on heat budget modeling. This ongoing effort, led by a Commission of the International Society of Biometeorology, has resulted in a proposed UTCI (Universal Thermal Climate Index; Jendritzky, 2002); there has been reasonable progress during the past three years. Thermal index development for humans generally remains focused, however, on assessment of comfort (in natural or built environments) and, to a lesser extent, on potential risks during extreme conditions, rather than on linkages to some measure of performance.

Indices for animals

Contrary to the focus of human-oriented thermal indices on comfort, the primary emphasis for domestic animals has been on indices to support rational environmental management decisions related to performance, health, and well-being (Hahn & McQuigg, 1970a; Hahn, 1976, 1995). Efforts have been made to develop indices based on heat exchange; however, a more useful approach has been to evaluate the animal responses to a "standard" index. This approach recognizes the ability of the animal to cope with environmental stressors. Animals are remarkable in their ability to cope with such stressors, and within limits, can adjust physiologically, behaviorally, and immunologically to minimize adverse effects (Hahn, 1999), or even compensate for reduced performance during moderate environmental challenges (Hahn, 1982). Only when the magnitude (intensity and duration) of potential stressors exceeds thresholds, coupled with limited opportunity for recovery, are animals unable to cope and affected adversely (Figure 1). Hahn (1989; 1999), Hahn et al. (1991),

---

[1] THI can be calculated from the following equations, where drybulb temperature (TDB), wetbulb temperature (TWB), and dewpoint temperature (TDP) are °C and relative humidity (RH) is %: THI = 0.72 (TDB + TWB) + 40.6; THI = TDB+ (0.36*TDP)+41.2; THI = ((TDB*1.8)+32)-((0.55*(RH/100)))*(((TDB*1.8)+32)-58.

DeDios & Hahn (1993), Brown-Brandl et al. (2002), and Brown-Brandl et al. (2003) have reported on the dynamics of thermoregulatory responses of animals to thermal challenges. Young & Hall (1996) and Young et al. (1997) have further recognized the dynamics of this situation in their "functional body heat content model."

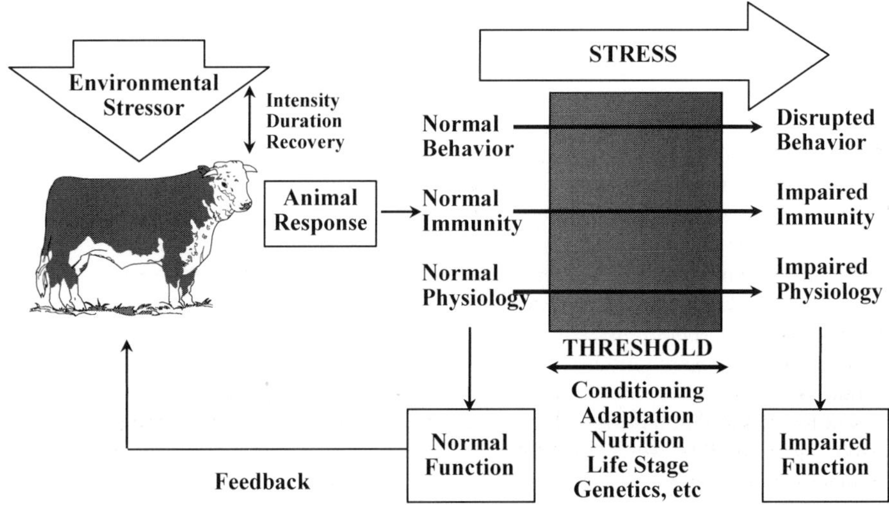

Figure 1. Responses of an animal to potential thermal stressors are complex, and can lead to reduced performance, health and well-being (adapted from Hahn and Becker, 1984; Hahn & Morrow-Tesch, 1993).

Indices based on heat exchange

Yamamoto (1983) provides a good discussion of the influence of humidity, air movement, and thermal radiation on heat exchanges related to effective temperatures. He concluded that "Heat exchanges between animals and their thermal environment are not [readily] explainable in terms of physical principles because the relationships are considerably modified [by] animal factors." In part, this reflects physiological differences among species in sensible and latent heat dissipation as they respond to the heat exchange parameters. These differences have been recognized in various indices that have been developed which are similar to the effective temperature (ET). Behavioral aspects (e.g., huddling in cold; wetting in heat) also can markedly alter heat exchanges.

A heat-exchange-based index for growing-finishing swine (typically 30-90 kg bodyweight) was experimentally determined by Roller & Goldman (1969), based on ambient drybulb (TDB) and wetbulb (TWB) temperatures (°C) for moderate conditions: Swine ET Index = 0.75TDB + 0.25TWB. For smaller swine (20-30 kg), Ingram (1965) found a slightly higher sensitivity to TWB, with the coefficients being 0.65 and 0.35 for TDB and TWB, respectively. A series of studies with poultry have determined coefficients for TDB/TWB: 0.60/0.40 for laying hens (Zulovich & DeShazer, 1990); 0.74/0.26 for 16-wk old hen turkeys (Xin et al., 1992); and 0.53/0.47 for 15-wk old tom turkeys (Brown-Brandl et al., 1997). Swine and poultry are basically non-sweating species, so that air moisture content has less influence than for species having a better ability to dissipate heat through skin vaporization.

For beef cattle, a species with more capabilities to dissipate latent heat through the skin, Bianca (1962) developed a relationship which indicates a greater sensitivity to air moisture content, with coefficients of 0.35 and 0.65 for TDB and TWB, respectively.
For cold-weather conditions, Ames & Insley (1975) developed wind-chill equations for cattle and sheep, which recognize the considerable effect of haircoat on heat exchange with the surroundings.

Indices-based response functions

Thermal indices have proven quite useful for environmental management of domestic animals through linkages with animal performance by means of biologic response functions (Hahn & McQuigg, 1970a; Hahn, 1976; Baccari, 2001). The linkage is based on observations of a selected performance criterion (e.g., growth, milk, or egg production) made concurrently with measures of the thermal environment as input for the selected thermal index, and an empirical relationship developed. This places more emphasis on the biological consequences associated with the index values. Additionally, if the same thermal index is selected for the response functions of multiple performance criteria and species, there is opportunity for broader application of the index climatology.
The Temperature-Humidity Index (THI) of Thom (1959) has been extensively applied for moderate to hot conditions using this approach, even with recognized limitations related to airspeed and radiation heat loads. In part, this is because temperature alone is usually inadequate for representing the overall thermal conditions, especially in outdoor environments. However, temperature and humidity do influence much of the heat exchange impacts of thermal environments, and hence often adequately represent the overall impact on livestock. At the latest International Livestock Environment Symposium (ILES, 2001), there were more than 15 articles that reported environmental conditions for animal studies or management (mostly for cattle, but some for poultry) in terms of the THI or a variant. At the present time, the THI has become a *de facto* standard for classifying thermal environments in many animal studies and selection of management practices during seasons other than winter.
The earliest example of the application of the THI as the basis for livestock response functions was for milk production decline (MDEC, kg/cow-day) of dairy cows, which was linked to the THI by means of the equation (Berry, et al., 1964):

$$MDEC = 1.075 - 1.736(NL) + 0.02474(NL)(THI)$$

where NL = normal level of milk production in thermoneutral conditions, kg/cow-day. This response function was developed through observations of responses of lactating dairy cows during exposure for several days to a selected regime of air temperatures and humidities while housed in environmental chambers (low airflow and nil radiation load [i.e., mean radiant temperature, MRT = air temperature]). The lower threshold THI for observed adverse effects on milk production is about 74, depending on the normal level of production (lower for high-producing cows and higher for low production levels).
A similar approach has been used to link the growth of broiler chickens to the THI (Ibrihim et al., 1975). Reproduction of dairy cows also has been linked to the THI based on field observations in Mexico and Hawaii (Ingraham et al, 1974).
Even with the obvious limitations on the THI-based MDEC response function for dairy cows (e.g., disregard of airflow and thermal radiation components of the environment), it has been successfully used in a variety of research studies and management applications. Initially, it was used to estimate milk production declines during summer months for shaded dairy cows in various U.S. locations, based on climatological analyses of the THI (Figure 2; Hahn & McQuigg, 1970b; Hahn & Osburn, 1969). These estimated production declines compared favorably (within 4-15%) with actual declines measured during summertime trials in four

divergent U.S. locations (Hahn, 1969). Other climatic analyses of the THI have since been completed for other U.S. locales (e.g., Huhnke et al., 2001) and for several other dairy production areas of the world, where summer conditions cause reductions in production and reproduction. Examples of the latter include Argentina (Valtorta et al., 1998; Casa & Ravelo, 2003), Australia (Davison et al., 1996), Brazil (da Silva, 2000), and South Africa (du Preez et al., 1990). The response function has also been subsequently used to estimate the benefits of environmental modification practices for shaded lactating cows, such as evaporative cooling (Hahn & Osburn, 1970).

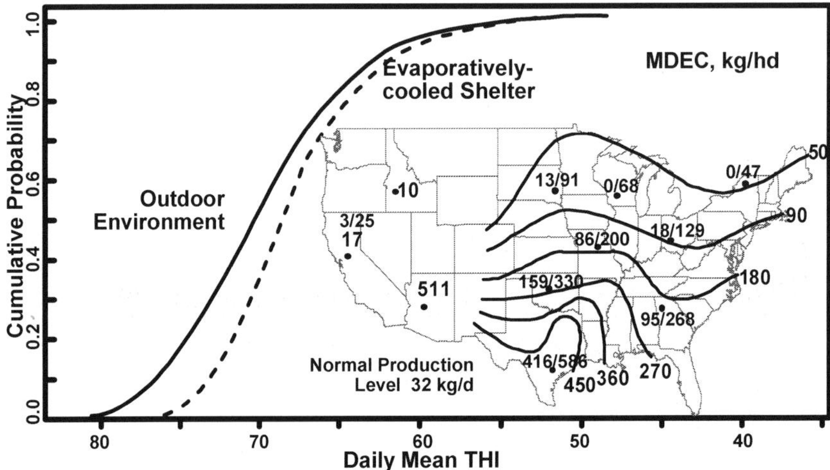

Figure 2. Probability distribution functions for daily mean THI in the naturally-varying outdoor environment and in evaporative-cooled shelters (Hahn and Osburn, 1970) at Columbia, MO during the June 1-Sept 30 summer season. The inset U.S. map shows associated expected milk production declines (MDEC) for dairy cows with a 32 kg/d normal production level (Hahn and McQuigg, 1970), along with 10 and 90 percentile values for selected locations (i.e., in central Missouri, 1 yr in 10 milk decline would be expected to be as low as 86 kg for the 122 day period, and 1 yr in 10 it would be as high as 200 kg [compared to the 180 kg average for that location]).

The THI has further been used as the basis for the Livestock Weather Safety Index (LWSI; LCI, 1970) to describe categories of heat stress associated with hot-weather conditions for livestock exposed to extreme conditions (Figure 3). The LWSI serves as a tactical guide for mitigating the effects of challenging environmental conditions on animals in intensive production systems, as well as during transport. For many years, the U.S. Agricultural Weather Advisory Service (AWAS) provided daily early-morning advisories when the LWSI was forecast to be in the Alert and higher categories, so that livestock personnel could plan to limit handling of animals and consider use of tactical measures to protect them. Since abolishment of the AWAS because of budgetary cutbacks in the U.S., some private weather services provide such advisories to subscribers for a fee. In New Zealand, the Meteorological Service currently provides heat stress forecasts for dairy cows <www.metservice.co.nz/data/hsigraph>.

Temperature, °C	Relative Humidity, %																			
	5	10	15	20	25	30	35	40	45	50	55	60	65	70	75	80	85	90	95	100
21	64	64	64	65	65	65	66	66	66	67	67	67	68	68	68	69	69	69	70	70
22	65	65	65	66	66	67	67	67	68	68	69	69	69	70	70	70	71	71	72	72
23	66	66	67	67	67	68	68	69	69	70	70	70	71	71	72	72	73	73	74	74
24	67	67	68	68	69	69	70	70	71	71	72	72	73	73	74	74	75	75	76	76
26	68	68	69	69	70	70	71	71	72	73	73	74	74	75	75	76	76	77	77	78
27	69	69	70	70	71	72	72	73	73	74	75	75	76	76	77	78	78	79	79	80
28	69	70	71	71	72	73	73	74	75	75	76	77	77	78	79	79	80	81	81	82
29	70	71	72	73	73	74	75	75	76	77	78	78	79	80	80	81	82	83	83	84
30	71	72	73	74	74	75	76	77	78	78	79	80	81	81	82	83	84	84	85	86
31	72	73	74	75	76	76	77	78	79	80	81	81	82	83	84	85	86	86	87	88
32	73	74	75	76	77	78	79	79	80	81	82	83	84	85	86	86	87	88	89	90
33	74	75	76	77	78	79	80	81	82	83	84	85	85	86	87	88	89	90	91	92
34	75	76	77	78	79	80	81	82	83	84	85	86	87	88	89	90	91	92	93	94
36	76	77	78	79	80	81	82	83	85	86	87	88	89	90	91	92	93	94	95	96
37	77	78	79	80	82	83	84	85	86	87	88	89	90	91	93	94	95	96	97	98
38	78	79	80	82	83	84	85	86	87	88	90	91	92	93	94	95	97	98	99	100
39	79	80	81	83	84	85	86	87	89	90	91	92	94	95	96	97	98	100	101	102
40	80	81	82	84	85	86	88	89	90	91	93	94	95	96	98	99	100	101	103	104
41	81	82	84	85	86	88	89	90	91	93	94	95	97	98	99	101	102	103	105	106
42	82	83	85	86	87	89	90	92	93	94	96	97	98	100	101	103	104	105	107	108
43	83	84	86	87	89	90	91	93	94	96	97	99	100	101	103	104	106	107	109	110

Categories of Livestock Weather Safety Index associated with THI values:
Normal: ≤ 74 Alert: 75-78 Danger: 79-83 Emergency: ≥84

Figure 3. Temperature-Humidity Index (THI) chart (based on Thom, 1959). Associated Livestock Weather Safety Index (LWSI; LCI, 1970) categories are also shown.

In connection with extreme conditions associated with heat waves, the THI has recently been used to evaluate spatial and temporal aspects of their development (Hubbard et al., 1999; Hahn & Mader, 1997). For cattle in feedlots, a THI-based classification scheme has also been developed to assess the potential impact of heat waves (Hahn et al., 1999). The classifications are based on a retrospective analysis of heat waves that have resulted in extensive feedlot cattle deaths, using a THI-hours approach[2] to assess the magnitude (intensity x duration) of the heat wave events which put the animals at risk.
Concerns with potential climate change impacts of animal agriculture have also led to the use of the THI for assessing such impacts on production and related measures. For example, the effects on milk production have been evaluated for either potential global cooling resulting from supersonic transport planes (Johnson et al., 1975) or current concerns about possible global warming associated with fossil fuel use and other human activities (Hahn et al., 1992; Klinedinst et al., 1993).

Modifications to the THI

Modifications to the THI have been proposed to overcome the shortcomings related to airflow and radiation heat loads. An example is the Black-Globe Temperature-Humidity Index (BGHI; Buffington et al., 1981), which uses black-globe temperature (Bond & Kelly, 1955)

[2] The daily THI-hrs were calculated from: $Daily\ THI\!-\!hrs = \sum_{hr=1}^{24} (THI - base)$.

instead of drybulb temperature in the THI equation. Applications of the BGHI to dairy cows suggested that values of 70 or below had little impact, while values of 75 or higher markedly reduce feed intake (Buffington et al., 1981); more recently, Buffington and others agree that a threshold of 75 for marked reduction in feed intake is likely too high given the current milk production levels, genetics, and use of bovine somatotropin (Gooch & Inglis, 2001).
Based on recent research, Mader & Davis (2002) and Eigenberg et al. (2002) have proposed corrections to the THI for use with feedlot cattle, based on measures of windspeed (WS) and solar radiation (SRAD). For a range of conditions from 25-40°C and 30-50% RH, the THI adjustments as evaluated by Mader & Davis (2002) were +2.7 for an increase in SRAD of 100 W/m^2, and -2.4 for a WS increase of 1m/s, based on panting scores of observed animals. Comparatively, the equivalent THI adjustments for the same increases in SRAD and WS, as determined by Eigenberg et al. (2002) from observations of respiration rate (RR), were +0.53 and -0.14, respectively, for the same range of conditions. While the proposed adjustment factor differences are substantial, there were marked differences in the types and number of animals used in the two studies. Nevertheless, the approach appears to merit further research to establish acceptable THI corrections, perhaps for a variety of animal parameters.

Other approaches to development of animal indices

Baeta et al. (1987) developed an Equivalent Temperature Index (ETI) for dairy cows in above-thermoneutral conditions, which combined the effects of air temperature and humidity with airspeed to evaluate the impacts on heat dissipation and milk production (Figure 4). So far, the ETI has not been widely accepted, perhaps because of the 3-day treatment observation periods. Nevertheless, it may provide representative results for short-term heat challenges that often occur in the summer season.
A somewhat similar approach was used to derive an Apparent Equivalent Temperature (AET) from air temperature and vapor pressure to develop "thermal comfort zones" for transport of broiler chickens (Mitchell et al., 2001). Experimental studies to link the AET with increased body temperature during exposure to hot conditions indicated potential for improved transport practices.
Gaughan et al. (2002) have developed a Heat Load Index (HLI) as a guide to management of unshaded Bos taurus feedlot cattle during hot weather (>28°C). The HLI was developed following observation of behavioral responses (RR and panting score) and changes in dry matter intake during prevailing thermal conditions. The HLI is based on humidity (RH, %), windspeed (WS, km/h), and predicted black globe temperature (PredTBG [°C], computed from air temperature [TDB, °C] and solar radiation [SRAD, w/m^2]):

$$HLI = 33.2 + 0.2RH + 1.2PredTBG - (0.82WS)^{0.1} - LOG10(0.4WS^2 + 0.0001)$$

where PredTBG is obtained by calculation[3]:

$$PredTBG = 1.33TDB - 2.65(TDB)^{1/2} + 3.21*LOG10(SRAD + 1) + 3.5.$$

During inital trials in 2002, the HLI was a good indicator of physiological stress on feedlot cattle, and has now been implemented as a heat load warning guide on the Internet <www.katestone.com.au/mla>, as both a current and 5-day forecast for Australian producers.
Using the approach that animals themselves provide an integrated response to their thermal environment, Eigenberg et al. (2002) also developed a linear regression-based estimator for RR of feedlot cattle at temperature levels above 25°C, using input parameters of TDB, RH, WS and SRAD (as defined above). The equations for shaded and unshaded animals, based on direct observations of RR, were:

[3] The original HLI equation was based on actual TBG; however, comparison of PredTBG with actual TBG showed R^2=0.9355, based on 9388 data points collected at four feedlots (E.A. Systems, 2002), so PredTBG is now used (John Gaughan, personal communication, 2003).

No Shade, TDB>25°C: RR = 5.4TDB + 0.58RH - 0.63WS + 0.024SRAD - 110.9
Shade, TDB>25°C: RR = 2.8TDB - 0.39RH + 0.36WS + 0.0064SRAD - 30.0
The RR estimator serves as the basis for alerting feedlot managers to possible thermal stress in their animals, and has been used to implement an environmental monitoring device for livestock production facilities (Eigenberg et al., 2003).

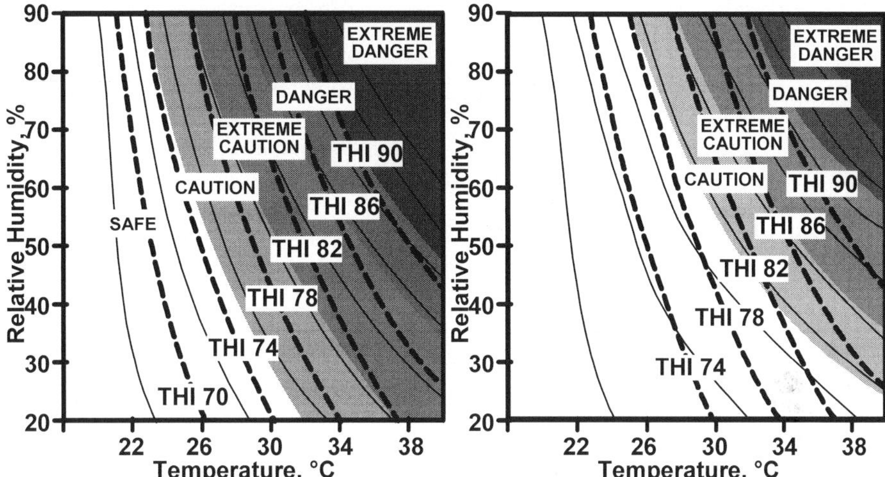

Figure 4. Equivalent Temperature Index (ETI) as a function of ambient temperature and humidity at windspeeds of 0.5 ms/ (left) and 6 m/s (right), with associated categories of potential impact on dairy cows (Baeta et al., 1987). Values of THI are superimposed for comparison.

Use of indices as a basis for environmental management of animals

Rational environmental management requires information about potential risks to the animals and to the production enterprise from thermal challenges. Three elements of risk need to be considered: 1) perception, 2) evaluation, and 3) management. Perception requires recognition of the potential threat from thermal conditions at the location of the animals, and can be at scales of the macro-environment (e.g., blizzards, heat waves) or the microenvironment (e.g., noxious gases in housing). Evaluation requires some assessment of the potential consequences from the perceived threat (e.g., likelihood of occurrence of adverse conditions and associated impacts on performance, health, and well-being of the animals; economic impact on the production enterprise). Management involves decisions, to accept the consequences or to take action to mitigate the potential effects.
The use of indices in support of environmental management decisions for livestock is needed at two levels: 1) to assess long-term climate impacts on the production system (strategic decisions), which recognize the ability of animals to acclimatize and compensate for short-term environmental challenges, and 2) to evaluate the near-term consequences of current weather (tactical decisions), which influence the day-to-day dynamics of thermoregulation and related responses. Examples of strategic decisions are those related to the need for buffered environments (e.g., housing, shades, windbreaks), both to protect and to maintain the productive function of the animals. Tactical decisions involve the use of available

environmental modification practices (e.g., sprinklers, fans, heaters), first as protective measures but also in support of the productive function.

As a result of its demonstrated broad success, the THI is currently the most widely-accepted thermal index used for guidance of strategic and tactical decisions in animal management during moderate to hot conditions. Biologic response functions, when combined with likelihood of occurrence of the THI for specific locations, provide the basis for economic evaluation to make cost-benefit comparisons for rational strategic decisions among alternatives (Hahn, 1981). Developing climatology of summer weather extremes (in particular, heat waves) for specific locations also provides the livestock manager with information about how often those extremes (with possible associated death losses) might occur (Hahn et al., 2001). The THI has also served well for tactical decisions on when to apply available practices and techniques (e.g., sprinkling) during either normal weather variability or weather extremes, such as heat waves.

Considerations for the future: what are the most potentially-useful approaches for further development of thermal indices for animals?

Does the success of the THI, particularly for cattle applications, mean it is the best thermal index that can be developed for all livestock applications? The answer is obvious--*NO!* This is primarily because of its limitations related to thermal radiation, airflow, and cold conditions; additionally, there are specie-specific limitations (e.g., non-sweating swine and poultry, which respond quite differently to warm environments than cattle). There are even limited cases where air temperature alone has been shown to be an adequate representation of the impact of hot thermal environments; in intensive animal housing with environmental modification, temperature alone is also the usual control parameter. However, the THI, by combining temperature and humidity effects, does capture much of the impact of warm to hot thermal environments on animals, especially in buffered environments (e.g., dairy cows and poultry protected from the direct effects of the naturally-varying weather). This suggests that the THI may remain a practical index for other than the winter season, and currently serves as the *de facto* standard for many livestock studies and applications, especially for cattle.

Nevertheless, efforts should continue for improving on the basic THI concept by incorporating the effects of thermal radiation and airflow, especially for animals in non-buffered moderate to hot environments and for animals in cold conditions. The substitution of black globe temperature for air temperature to obtain the BGHI (Buffington et al., 1981) appears to be useful in some applications, and adding modifiers to the THI to recognize thermal radiation and wind effects on animals in non-buffered environments (as suggested for feedlot cattle: Mader & Davis, 2002; Eigenberg et al., 2001) may have promise. The Heat Load Index (Gaughan et al., 2002), which uses predicted black globe temperature as a basic input, is currently undergoing further testing. Other approaches, such as the Apparent Equivalent Temperature proposed by Mitchell et al. (2001) for use in poultry transport, also may be appropriate. Enthalpy has been suggested as an alternative thermal index by Beckett (1965) for swine, and by Moura et al. (1997) for swine and poultry.

The success of THI-based environmental management for livestock, as outlined in the preceding section, lies not in the THI being the best possible thermal index, but in the development of biologic response functions which link important animal responses to the THI. Relationships for long-term strategic decisions (e.g., evaluating the need for and selection of economical environmental modification practices) must recognize the ability of animals to acclimatize during long-term exposure to challenging thermal environments. Response relationships useful for short-term tactical decisions (day-to-day operations, such as handling practices and use of heating/cooling equipment), must recognize the dynamics of the animal response to short-term environmental challenges. The outcome of current applications of this dual approach, even with the limitations of current information, has been improved production, health, and well-being of animals in adverse climates, especially during weather extremes.

Any modified or replacement index must be pragmatic in the face of limited resources available for development and application. Regardless of the level of sophistication, thermal indices need to be developed in a way that improves on the foundation of applications that have served livestock managers well in their decision-making process. That means any improved index will ideally be useful as a basis for continued development of biologic response functions, and representative of the consequences resulting from primary factors influencing energy exchanges between the animal and its surroundings. For strategic decision-making, a proliferation of indices, each with limited application, is not recommended--the goal should be an index that is broadly applicable across life stages and species, in order to maximize the utility of probability information about the index. For tactical decisions, modifiers for primary indices and/or specialty indices which focus more on immediate physiological responses of the animals to heat exchanges with the thermal environment may be appropriate. An alternative for tactical decisions is observation of the animals themselves as an integrator of the impact of the thermal environment (Young et al., 1997; Eigenberg, et al., 2002).

Acknowledgements

The authors gratefully acknowledge the past influence and guidance of many colleagues around the world who have contributed in one way or another, to the discussions presented here. Rather than attempt to recognize anyone specifically, we thank all those who are past and present participants in the Congresses of the International Society of Biometeorology (ISB) and the International Commission of Agricultural Engineering (CIGR); Symposia of the European Association of Animal Production (EAAP), the American Society of Agricultural Engineers (ASAE), the American Society of Animal Science (ASAS); and other similar conferences which have provided the foundation for progress in this area.

References

Ames, D.A. & L.W. Insley. 1975. Wind-chill effect for cattle and sheep. J. Anim. Sci. 40(1): 161-165

Baccari, Flavio, Jr. 2001. Manejo ambiental da vacaleiteira em climas quentes. Editora da Universidade Estadual de Londrina. Londrina PR-Brazil (142 pp).

Baeta, F.C., N.F. Meador, M.D. Shanklin & H.D. Johnson. 1987. Equivalent temperature index at temperatures above the thermoneutral for lactating dairy cows. Paper No. 87-4015, Am. Soc. Ag. Eng., St. Joseph, MI.

Beckett, F.E., 1965. Effective temperature for evaluating or designing hog environments. Trans. ASAE 8(2): 163-166.

Berry, I.L., M.D. Shanklin & H.D. Johnson, 1964. Dairy shelter design based on milk production decline as affected by temperature and humidity. Trans. ASAE 7(3): 329-331.

Bianca, W., 1962. Relative importance of dry- and wet-bulb temperatures in causing heat stress in cattle. Nature 195: 251-252.

Bond, T.E. & C.F. Kelly, 1955. The globe thermometer in agricultural research. Agric. Eng. 36: 251-255, 260.

Brown-Brandl, T.M., M.M. Beck, D.D. Schulte, A.M. Parkhurst & J.A. DeShazer, 1997. Temperature-Humidity Index for growing tom turkeys. Trans. ASAE 49)1):203-209.

Brown-Brandl, T.M., R.A. Eigenberg, G.L. Hahn, J.A. Nienaber, T.L. Mader, D.E. Spiers & A.M. Parkhurst, 2002. Dynamic responses of feeder cattle to simulated heat waves. Paper Number 024051, Am. Soc. Ag. Eng., St Joseph MI.

Brown-Brandl, T.M., J.A. Nienaber, R.A. Eigenberg, G.L. Hahn & H. Freetly, 2003. Thermoregulatory responses of feeder cattle. J. Therm. Biol. 28: 149-157.

Buffington, D.E., A. Collazon-Arocho, G.H. Canton & D. Pitt, 1981. Black globe-humidity index (BGHI) as comfort equation for dairy cows. Trans. ASAE 24(3): 711-714.

da Silva, R.G. 2000. Introducao a bioclimatologia animal. Nobel, Sao Paulo, Brazil. 286 pp

Davison, T., M. McGowan, D. Mayer, B. Young, N. Jonsson, A. Hall, A. Matschoss, P. Goodwin, J. Gaughan & M. Lake, 1996. Managing hot cows in Australia. QDPI, Brisbane 4001, Australia

De Dios, O.O. & G.L. Hahn, 1993. Thermoregulation of growing bovines during fall transitional environments. Proc 4th Intl. Lvstk. Environ. Symp.: 289-297.

de la Casa, A. & A.C. Ravelo, 2003. Assessing temperature and humidity conditions for dairy cattle in Cordoba, Argentina. Int'l. J. Biomet. (in press)

du Preez, J.H., W.H. Giesecke & P.J. Hattingh, 1990. Heat stress in dairy cattle and other livestock under southern African conditions. I. Temperature- Humidity Index mean values during the four main seasons. Onderstepoort J. Vet. Res. 57: 77-87.

E.A. Systems P/L, 2002. Measuring the microclimate of Eastern Australia feedlots. Final report for project FLOT.317, MLA, Sydney NSW, Australia. pp 40-44.

Eigenberg, R.A., T.M. Brown-Brandl, J.A. Nienaber & G.L. Hahn, 2002. Dynamic response of feedlot cattle to shade and no-shade. Paper No. 024050, Am. Soc. Ag. Eng., St Joseph MI.

Eigenberg, R.A., J.A.Nienaber & T.M. Brown-Brandl, 2003. Development of a livestock safety monitor for cattle. Paper No. 032338. Am. Soc. Ag. Eng., St Joseph MI.

Gaughan, J.G., J. Goopy & J. Spark. 2002. Excessive heat load index for feedlot cattle. Meat and Livestock-Australia Project Rept, FLOT.316. MLA, Ltd., Locked Bag 991, N. Sydney NSW, 2059 Australia.

Gooch, C.A. & S.F. Inglis, 2001. Environmental conditions in plastic film covered calf facilities. Proc. 6th Intl Lvstk Environ Symp, Am. Soc. Ag. Eng., St Joseph MI. pp 703-715

Hahn, G.L., 1969. Predicted vs. measured production differences using summer air conditioning for lactating dairy cows. J. Dairy Sci. 52(6): 800-802.

Hahn, G.L., 1976. Rational environmental planning for efficient livestock production. Biomet. 6 (Part II): 106-114.

Hahn, G.L., 1981. Housing and management to reduce climatic impacts on livestock. J. Ani. Sci. 52(1): 175-186.

Hahn, G.L., 1982. Compensatory performance in livestock: influences on environmental criteria. Proc. 2nd Int'l. Lvstk. Environ. Symp., ASAE SP-03-82. Am. Soc. Ag. Eng., St Joseph, MI. pp 285-294.

Hahn, G.L., 1989. Body temperature rhythms in farm animals--a review and reassessment relative to environmental influences. Proc., 11th Int'l. Soc. Biomet. Congress, West Lafayette, IN. pp. 325-337.

Hahn, G.L., 1995. Environmental management for improved livestock performance, health and well-being. Japanese Jour. Lvstk. Mgt. 30(3): 113-127.

Hahn, G.L., 1999. Dynamic responses of cattle to thermal heat loads. J. Anim. Sci. 77 (Suppl. 2): 10-20.

Hahn, G.L. & B.A. Becker, 1984. Assessing livestock stress. Agric. Engr. 65(11): 15-17.

Hahn, G.L., Y.R. Chen, J.A. Nienaber, R.A. Eigenberg & A.M. Parkhurst, 1991. Characterizing animal stress through fractal analysis of thermoregulatory responses. J. Thermal Biol. 17(2): 115-120.

Hahn, G.L., P.L. Klinedinst & D.A. Wilhite, 1992. Climate change impacts on livestock production and management. ASAE Paper 927037. Am. Soc. Ag. Eng., St Joseph MI.

Hahn, G.L. & T.L Mader, 1997. Heat waves in relation to thermoregulation, feeding behavior and mortality of feedlot cattle. Proc. 5th Int'l. Lvstk. Environ. Symp. ASAE SP01-97, Am. Soc. Ag. Eng., St Joseph MI. (Vol. I): pp. 563-571.

Hahn, G.L., T.L. Mader, J.B. Gaughan, Q. Hu & J.A. Nienaber, 1999. Heat waves and their impacts on feedlot cattle. Proc. 15th Int'l. Cong. of Biomet. and Int'l. Cong. on Urban Climatology:, Sydney, Australia.

Hahn, L., T. Mader, D. Spiers, J. Gaughan, J. Nienaber, R. Eigenberg, T. Brown-Brandl, Q. Hu, D. Griffin, L. Hungerford, A. Parkhurst, M. Leonard, W. Adams & L. Adams, 2001. Heat wave impacts on feedlot cattle: considerations for improved environmental management. Proc. 6th Int'l. Lvstk. Environ. Symp.: Am. Soc. Agric. Eng., St. Joseph, MI. pp. 129-139.

Hahn, L. & J.D. McQuigg, 1970a. Expected production losses for lactating Holstein dairy cows as a basis for rational planning of shelters. Int'l. J. Farm Bldgs. Res. 4: 2-8.

Hahn, L. & J.D. McQuigg, 1970b. Evaluation of climatological records for rational planning of livestock shelters. Ag. Met. 7(2): 131-141.

Hahn, G.L. & J.L. Morrow-Tesch. 1993. Improving livestock care and well-being. Ag Eng 74(3): 14-17.

Hahn, G.L. & D.D. Osburn, 1969. Feasibility of summer environmental control for dairy cattle based on expected production losses. Trans. Am. Soc. Agric. Eng. 12(4): 448-451.

Hahn, L. & D.D. Osburn, 1970. Feasibility of evaporative cooling for dairy cattle based on expected production losses. Trans. Am. Soc. Agric. Eng. 13(3): 289-291, 294.

Hahn, G.L. 1995. Environmental management for improved livestock performance, health and well-being. Japanese J. Lvstk. Mgt. 30(3):113-127

Hendrick, R.L. 1959. An outdoor weather-comfort index for the summer season in Hartford, Connecticut. Bull. Am. Met. Soc. 40: 620-623.

Houghten, F.C. & C.P. Yaglou. 1923. Determination of the comfort zone. Trans. Am. Soc. of Heating and Ventilating Engrs. 29: 361-384.

Houghton, D.D. (editor). 1985. Handbook of Applied Meteorology. John Wiley and Sons, New York, (589pp).

Hubbard, K.G., D.E. Stooksbury, G.L. Hahn & T.L. Mader, 1999. A climatological perspective on feedlot cattle performance and mortality related to the temperature-humidity index. J. Prod. Agric. 12: 650-653.

Huhnke, R.L., L.C.McCowan, G.M. Meraz, S.L. Harp & M.E. Payton. 2001. Determining the frequency and duration of elevated Temperature-Humidity Index. Tech. Rept. No. 01-4111, Am. Soc. Ag. Eng., St Joseph, MI.

Ibrahim, M.N, D.G. Stevens, M.D. Shanklin & L. Hahn, 1975. Model of broiler performance as affected by temperature and humidity. Trans. ASAE, 18(5): 960-962.

ILES 6, 2001. Livestock Environment VI. Proc., 6th Int'l. Lvstk. Environ. Symp., R.R. Stowell, R. Bucklin, R.W. Bottcher (eds.) Public. 701P0201, Am. Soc. Agric. Eng., St. Joseph, MI 763 pp.

Ingram, D.L., 1965. The effect of humidity on temperature regulation and cutaneous water loss in the young pig. Res. Vet Sci. 6(1): 9-17.

Ingraham, R.H., D.D. Gillette & W.D. Wagner, 1974. Relationship of temperature and humidity to conception rate of Holstein cows in subtropical climate. J. Dairy Sci. 57: 476-481.

Jendritzky, G., A. Maarouf, D. Fiala & H. Staiger. 2002. An update on the development of a Universal Thermal Climate Index. Proc. 15th AMS Conf. on Biomet. and Aeriobiology/16th Int'l. Cong. Biomet. AMS, Boston, MA. (USA), 129-133.

Johnson, H.D., L. Hahn & D.E. Buffington, 1975. Animal husbandry implications. Sect. 4.3, Chapt. 4, Agricultural Implications of Climatic Change, In: CIAP Monograph 5, Impacts of Climate Change on the Biosphere (Final Report). Climatic Impact Assessment Program (Stratospheric Pollution by Aircraft), Dept. of Transportation. 423 pp.

Klinedinst, P.L., D.A. Wilhite, G.L. Hahn & K.G. Hubbard, 1993. The potential effects of climate change on summer season dairy cattle milk production and reproduction. Climate Change 23: 21-36.

LCI, 1970. Patterns of transit losses. Livestock Conservation, Inc., Omaha, NE.

Mader, T.L., & M.S. Davis, 2002. Wind speed and solar radiation correction for the Temperature-Humidity Index. Proc. 16th Cong. Int'l. Soc. Biomet./15th Am. Met. Soc. Conf. Biomet. and Aerobiol. Boston, MA. pp 154-157.

Mitchell, M.A., P.J. Kettlewell, R.R. Hunter & A.J. Carlisle, 2001. Physiological stress response modeling--applications to the broiler transport thermal environment. Proc. 6th Int'l Lvstk. Environ. Symp., Am. Soc. Agric. Eng., St Joseph MI. pp 550-555.

Moura, D.J., I.A. Naas, K.B. Sevegnani & M.E. Corria, 1997. The use of enthalpy as a thermal comfort index. Proc. 5th Int'l. Lvstk. Environ. Symp., Am. Soc. Agric. Eng., St. Joseph, MI. pp 577-583.

Roller, W.L. & R.F. Goldman, 1969. Response of swine to acute heat exposure. Trans. Am. Soc. Ag. Engr. 12(2): 164-169, 174.

Siple, P.A. & C.F. Passel, 1945. Measurements of dry atmospheric cooling in subfreezing temperatures. Proc. Amer. Phil. Soc. 89: 177-199.

Thom, E.C, 1959. The Discomfort Index. Weatherwise 12: 57-60.

Valtorta, S., P. Leva, H. Castro, M. Gallardo, M. Maciel, A. Guglielmone & O, Anziani, 1998. Produccion de lecha en verano, page 18. Universidad Nacional del Litoral, Santa Fe, Argentina. 105 pp.

Watts, J.D. & L.S. Kalkstein, 2002. The development of a warm-weather relative comfort index for environmental analysis. Proc. 15th Conf on Biomet. and Aerobiology/16th Int'l. Cong. on Biomet.: 126-128.

Xin, H., J.A. DeShazer & M.M. Beck, 1992. Responses of pre-fasted growing turkeys to acute heat exposure. Trans. ASAE 35(1): 315-318.

Yamamoto, S., 1983. The assessment of thermal environment for farm animals. Proc. 5th World Cong. Animal Prod., Vol 1: 197-204.

Young, B.A. & A.B. Hall, 1996. Thermal environment and heat prostration in farm animals. 8th AAAP Anim. Sci. Cong. (Japan) 1: 555-560.

Young, B.A., A.B. Hall, P.J. Goodwin & J.B. Gaughan, 1997. Identifying excessive heat load. Proc. 5th Int'l. Symp. Lvstk. Environ, Am. Soc. Ag. Eng., St. Joseph, MI. pp. 572-576.

Zulovich, J.M. & J.A. DeShazer, 1990. Estimating egg production declines at high environmental temperatures and humidities. Paper No. 90-4021, Am. Soc. Ag. Eng., St. Joseph, MI.

Physiological and productive consequences of heat stress. The case of dairy ruminants

N. Lacetera, U. Bernabucci, B. Ronchi & A. Nardone

Dipartimento di Produzioni Animali, Via De Lellis, 01100 Viterbo, Italy, nicgio@unitus.it

Summary

This paper reviews and discusses physiological and productive consequences of heat stress (HS) in high yielding and intensively managed dairy ruminants. As for other homeothermic animals, HS in dairy ruminants is characterised by adaptive changes of physiological functions in the attempt to avoid hyperthermia. In turn, such changes and/or hyperthermia cause modifications of non-adaptive physiological functions, reproduction, growth, lactation, milk quality, and health, which have been studied extensively only in dairy cows. In dairy cows HS reduces conception rate, increases embryo mortality, impairs luteal function, disturbs gonadotrophin and oestradiol secretions, modifies oestrus expression and follicular dynamics, and increases the frequency of silent oestrus and development of ovarian cysts. When dairy heifers suffer from HS daily gain is lowered, gross efficiency of converting nutrients to tissue is reduced, and biometric parameters change. In dairy cows, sheep, goats and water buffaloes HS reduces milk yield. Exposure to high ambient temperatures (HAT) modifies also milk and colostrum composition. Results on the effects of HS on milk fat in dairy cows are conflicting. In dairy sheep exposure to solar radiation reduces milk fat yield. Milk and colostrum from heat stressed dairy cows have less protein and lactose, higher pH, and lower titratable acidity. Lactose concentration decreases in goats' milk after exposure to HAT. Milk yielded from heat stressed cows has lower calcium, phosphorous and magnesium, higher chloride and freezing point. Milk and colostrum from heat stressed dairy cows has low proportions of short (C_4-C_{10}) and medium-chain (C_{12}-C_{16}) fatty acids (FAA), and high proportions of long-chain (C_{17}-C_{18n}) FAA. In dairy sheep exposure to solar radiation reduces proportions of mono- and polyunsaturated FAA and increased those of C_{12}-C_{16} FAA. Milk from summer cows has lower α_s and β-caseins, lower casein number, and higher milk serum proteins. Conversely, HAT do not modify α-lactalbumin and β-lactoglobulin concentrations of bovine milk. Exposure of dairy sheep to solar radiation reduces casein yield. Results on the effects of HAT on protective value of bovine colostrum are conflicting. Exposure of sheep to solar radiation also worsens the hygienic quality of milk. Exposure to HAT can modify the incidence of parasitic diseases and cause death losses. Whether metabolic changes, pro-oxidant antioxidant balance, and changes of the immune functions represent HS-related phenomena that can modify health of intensively managed dairy ruminants is discussed.

Keywords: ruminants, heat stress, reproduction, growth, lactation, health

Introduction

The ability of livestock to breed, grow, and lactate to their maximal genetic potential, and their capacity to maintain health is strongly affected by the thermal environment.

As for other homeothermic animals, when temperature humidity index (THI) is above the upper critical THI, ruminants avoid the hyperthermia by increasing heat loss and/or decreasing heat production (Johnson, 1987). As reviewed elsewhere, the ability of ruminants to control body temperatures varies with species and breeds (Silanikove, 2000). However, despite species and breed, dissipation of heat is obtained by non-evaporative or sensible heat loss (conduction, convection and radiation) and evaporative water loss (cutaneous and respiratory) (Johnson, 1987). Reduction of heat production is achieved by reducing the energy transformations taking place in the animal per unit of time (Yousef, 1987). The immediate response of animals to high air temperature (HAT) is reduced feed intake, to attempt bringing metabolic heat production in line with heat dissipation capabilities. If the exposure to HAT is prolonged, the reduced feed intake is followed by hormonal changes and decline of metabolic rate and enzymatic activities (Webster, 1983).

All the events activated to avoid the hyperthermia or the hyperthermia itself contribute to the alterations of reproduction (Wolfenson et al., 2000), growth (Johnson, 1987), lactation (West et al., 2003), and health (Webster et al., 1983; Silanikove, 2000; Kadzere et al., 2002). These alterations have been widely documented in dairy cows, whereas experimental data referred to other dairy ruminants are limited.

This paper reviews and discusses some of the physiological and productive consequences of heat stress (HS) in high yielding and intensively managed dairy ruminants. Due to the already mentioned scarcity of information referred to other dairy ruminant species, namely sheep, goats and buffaloes, the majority of data reviewed and discussed herein are referred to dairy cows, and particular emphasis is given to the effects of HAT on milk quality and health.

Reproduction

Heat stress has been associated with reduction of reproductive efficiency due to a variety of factors (Johnson, 1987). The effects of the thermal environment on reproduction may take place through a direct action of the hyperthermia upon the reproductive tissues or through an indirect and subtler manner (lower nutrients intake, impairment of hypothalamic, pituitary, gonadal and endometrial secretions, redistribution of blood flow among body organs, etc.) (Wolfenson et al., 2000).

The most dramatic effects of HS on reproduction of dairy cows are represented by reduced conception rate (Wise et al., 1988), increased embryo mortality (Gwazdauskas et al., 1985; Paula-Lopes et al., 2003), impaired luteal function (Wolfenson et al., 1993; Ronchi et al., 2001), and disturbances in gonadotrophin (Gilad et al., 1993) and oestradiol (Wilson et al., 1998) secretions. In dairy cows HAT are also known to modify oestrus expression (Gwazdauskas et al., 1985) and follicular dynamics (Wilson et al., 1998), and to increase the frequency of silent oestrus (Rodtian et al., 1996). Moreover, Holstein cows calving in summer are 2.6 times more likely to develop ovarian cysts than those giving birth in winter (Lopez-Gatius et al., 2002).

Growth

When growing animals suffer from HS average daily gain is lowered and gross efficiency of converting nutrients to tissue is reduced (Ames et al., 1980). Furthermore, HS also affects body composition (NRC, 1981) and biometric parameters of growing heifers (Lacetera et al., 1994).

Exposure of pregnant dairy cows to HAT influences growth and development of the foetus (Collier et al., 1982).

The effects of HS on growing dairy heifers were illustrated by Baccari et al. (1983). They observed increase of body temperature, reduced feed intake, growth rate, plasma triiodothyronine and growth hormone. Young Holstein heifers (160 ± 20 days) exposed to HAT grow 25% less than a counterpart kept in thermoneutrality (Nardone et al., 1993), and show significant reductions of body capacity and impairment of growth of anatomical parts important for parturition and development of the udder (Lacetera et al., 1994).

Milk yield

In dairy cows HS is associated with a decline of milk yield (Bianca, 1965; Johnson, 1987; Bernabucci & Calamari, 1998). Johnson (1987) reviewed that milk yield declines when the environmental temperatures exceed 22-23°C. Previously, Johnson et al. (1962) showed a linear reduction of milk yield when THI exceeds 70: -0.26 kg/day/ unit of THI. However, the majority of researchers indicated 25°C as the upper critical temperature (NRC, 1981), and 72 as the upper critical THI (Armstrong, 1994) for lactating dairy cows. Recently, other authors indicated 68 as the upper critical THI in high yielding dairy cows (Ravagnolo & Misztal, 2002). In a study carried out in primiparous Holstein cows it was found that for each increase of 1 °C of the rectal temperature above physiological body temperature milk production declined 2.2 litres/day (Nardone et al., 1992). Similar results have been reported recently by Barash et al. (2001) in Israeli Holstein cows.

McDowell et al. (1969) proposed that reduced feed intake accounts for about 50 percent of the reduced milk yield. Remaining 50 % might depend on a heat-related decline of lactogenic hormones (Collier et al., 1982; Johnson et al., 1988b) and increase of maintenance requirements (NRC, 1981).

However, the extent of milk yield decline observed in heat stressed cows depends on a series of factors (i.e. breed, individual, yielding capacity, stage of lactation, feeding) that interact with HAT (Bernabucci & Calamari, 1998). High yielding cows are more sensitive to heat than low yielding cows, and equations to estimate milk loss in relation with yielding capacity and THI values have been proposed (Linvill & Pardue, 1992). Stage of lactation also affects response of dairy cows to HAT. Johnson et al. (1988a) observed that the mid-lactating dairy cows were the most heat sensitive compared to early or late lactating counterparts. Accordingly, studies carried out in climatic chambers described an HS-related decrease in milk yield of 35% in mid lactating (Nardone et al., 1992), and of 14% in early lactating dairy cows (Lacetera et al., 1996). Variations of nutritional-metabolic conditions during lactation might explain the higher sensitivity to HAT of mid lactating dairy cows. In fact, milk yield in early lactation is strongly supported by tissue stores mobilisation (lipid in particular) and less by feed intake, whereas milk yield in mid lactation is mostly supported by feed intake (Webster, 1987). Since metabolic utilisation of tissue stores has a higher efficiency compared to the metabolic utilisation of feed (Moe et al., 1971), the early lactating cows are expected to produce less metabolic heat per kg of milk yield, than mid lactating cows.

Exposure of lactating ewes to solar radiation under HAT reduced milk yield up to 20% respect to a counterpart provided with shade (Sevi et al., 2001).

Lactating goats exposed to moderate or severe hot for 4 d reduce milk yields by 3 and 13%, respectively (Sano et al., 1985).

Water buffaloes calving in summer yield significant less milk than buffaloes giving birth during other seasons (Catillo et al., 2002).

Milk quality

Exposure of dairy cows to HAT determines also significant modification of milk quality (Bianca, 1965; Bernabucci & Calamari, 1998).

Results on the effects of HS on milk fat percentages are conflicting (Nardone et al., 1992; Armstrong, 1994; Lacetera et al., 1996). Milk and colostrum from heat stressed cows present lower percentages of protein, and lactose, higher pH, and lower titratable acidity (Bianca, 1965; Nardone et al., 1997; Bernabucci & Calamari, 1998). Milk from summer cows presents also an impairment of rheological behaviour during cheese manufacturing and cheese yield (Calamari & Mariani, 1998). In a recent study it was reported that in Israeli Holstein dairy cows average milk protein production was reduced by 0.01 kg/°C (Barash et al., 2001). Milk yielded under HAT also has lower calcium, phosphorous and magnesium, and higher pH, chloride, and freezing point (Kume et al., 1989; Mariani et al., 1993; Bernabucci & Calamari, 1998).

In sheep, Sevi et al. (2001) reported that declines of milk yield due to the exposure to solar radiation causes also a decline of fat yields.

The lactose concentration of goats' milk decreased after 4 d of exposure to severe hot (Sano et al., 1985).

In sheep it has been also reported that the exposure to solar radiation has detrimental effects on the hygienic quality of milk consisting of high number of pathogens and polymorphonuclear leukocytes (Sevi et al., 2001).

A limited number of studies reviewed below documented that HAT can also affect fatty acids (FAA) composition and protein fractions of colostrum and milk from dairy cows or sheep. These aspects are of interest because of the strict relationships between FAA and protein compositions and technological and/or nutritional properties of colostrum or milk.

Milk fatty acids

In 1965 Bianca reported lower content of short-chain FAA and higher content of C_{16} and C_{18} in milk from heat stressed cows. Gallacier et al. (1974) and Palmquist et al. (1993) observed lower proportions of short-chain and higher proportions of long-chains FAA during warm months. Piva et al. (1993) found an increase of unsaturated FAA in milk yielded during summer months. None of these authors attributed changes of milk fatty acids to a direct effect of HS, and suggested that they had to be attributed to the higher dietary intake of fat or to the lower forage intake which usually occur during summer (Gallacier et al., 1974; Palmquist et al., 1993), or to a more massive utilisation of body reserves (Piva et al., 1993).

In a study carried out in climate chambers (Ronchi et al., 1995) it was also observed that milk from heat stressed dairy cows had low proportions of short (C_4-C_{10}) and medium-chain (C_{12}-C_{16}) FAA, and high proportions of long-chain (C_{17}-C_{18n}) FAA. In the same study heat stressed cows also yielded 25% less milk with a lower percentage of fat than their counterparts kept in thermal comfort. As a consequence of the different FAA composition of milk and of the different fat and milk yield, the daily production of milk FAA in cows exposed to HAT was lower with regard to short and medium-chain FAA and nearly the same with regard to long-chain FAA (Figure 1). Therefore, this results indicated that the higher proportion of long-chain FAA observed in milk from heat stressed cows had to be attributed to the reduced synthesis of short- and medium-chain FAA in the mammary gland cells rather than to a higher incorporation of long-chain FAA. It was hypothesised that the energy deficit status that characterises HS might be the cause for the lower synthesis of short and medium-chain FAA synthesised into the mammary gland (Smith et al., 1983). Moreover, it was also suggested that the higher availability of long-chain FAA coming from lipomobilization would not hesitate in their higher incorporation into milk because these FAA might utilised as energy sources by the mammary gland cells (Smith et al., 1983). All this would authorize to indicate that fat intake, changes in the pattern of feeding and/or lipid mobilisation would not represent the only factors affecting milk FAA changes in summer milk.

Accordingly, Nardone et al. (1997) reported an increase of long-chain and a reduction of short-chain FAA also in colostrum yielded by heat stressed heifers.

In contrast, a single study referred to dairy sheep (Sevi et al., 2002) documented that the exposure to solar radiation was responsible for a worsening of the nutritional properties of milk associated with changes of the FAA profile and consisting of a reduced proportions of mono- and polyunsaturated FAA and increased proportions of the C_{12}-C_{16} FAA, which are known to exert hypercolesterolaemic effects in humans.

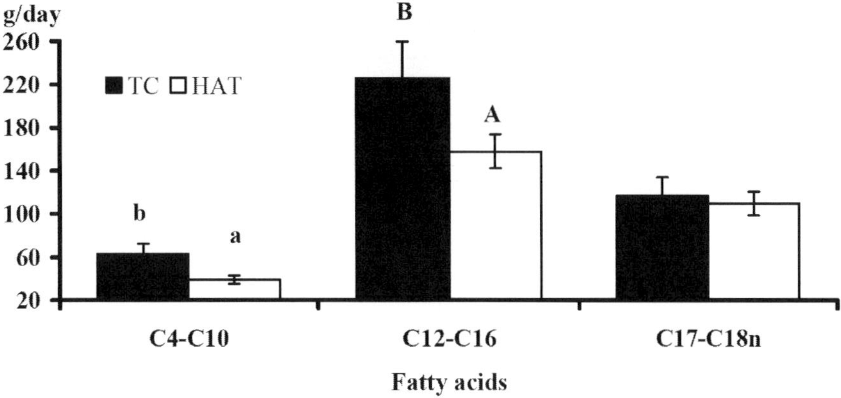

Figure 1. Lsmeans ± SE of milk short (C_4-C_{10}), medium (C_{12}-C_{16}) and long-chain (C_{17}-C_{18}) fatty acids (g/day) in Holstein cows exposed to thermal comfort (TC) and high ambient temperatures (HAT) (Ronchi et al., 1995).
abColumns with different letters differ significantly ($P<0.05$)
ABColumns with different letters differ significantly ($P<0.01$)

Milk protein fractions

The effects of HS on milk protein fractions have not been described extensively, and such lack of knowledge is surprising in the light of severe alterations of the cheesemaking properties of milk, reduction of cheese yield and alteration of cheese quality occurring in summer months around the world (Urech & Puhan, 1992; Ozimek & Kennelly, 1994; Mariani et al., 1995; Sevi et al., 2001).

Some authors reported a reduction of casein content in milk from summer cows (Hermansen et al., 1999; Mackle et al., 1999). In a previous study it was also observed lower casein content of colostrum from cattle exposed to HAT during the last three weeks of pregnancy (Nardone et al., 1997).

In a recent field study (Bernabucci et al., 2002a) we found that, compared to milk yielded from spring cows, summer milk had lower contents of crude proteins and caseins, lower casein number, and higher milk serum proteins (Table 1). Among caseins, the k-casein fraction did not differ between summer and spring cows. Conversely, milk from summer cows had lower of α_s- and β-caseins. In practice, results from this study indicated that the reduction of milk protein observed in summer was due to the reduction in the casein content, which was in turn caused by a reduction in α_s- and β-casein. The α_s- and β-casein represent approximately 90% of total caseins, contain a high numbers of phosphate groups (Schmidt, 1980), and their phosphorylation needs the presence of the γ-phosphate of ATP (Mercier & Gaye, 1983). This phosphorylation is significantly impaired under energy deficit conditions (Mackle et al., 1999), so that it has been hypothesised that the lower content of α_s- and β-casein in summer milk might be at least partially due to the reduction in energy and protein availability consequent to HS (Lacetera et al., 1996; Nardone et al., 1997). These changes might also explain the documented summer-related losses in cheese yield and alteration of cheesemaking properties (Urech & Puhan, 1992; Mariani et al., 1995; Ozimek & Kennelly, 1994). Moreover, α_s- and β-casein, rich in phosphate groups, are the two acidic components of the casein micelles (Schmidt, 1980). Thus, the lower contents of α_s- and β-casein of milk yielded during the summer might also explain the higher milk pH and the lower milk titratable acidity commonly recorded during hot summer months (Bernabucci & Calamari, 1998). Finally, the lower α_s- and β-casein contents might explain the lower milk phosphorous content observed by others (Forar et al., 1982; Kume et al., 1989) in milk yielded from cows exposed to HAT.

In the same study, we did not find seasonal variations of α-lactalbumin and β-lactoglobulin concentrations, even if serum proteins increased. Before our study, Hermansen et al. (1999) had already reported a higher content of whey proteins in milk produced in the late summer with indications that their result was not related to proteolysis. Since our result was not concomitant with mammary gland health problems, we hypothesised, according to Mackle et al. (1999), that it might be dependent on milk concentration due to decline of milk volume.

Table 1. Protein fractions (%) in milk from summer (SU) and spring (SP) cows (Bernabucci et al., 2002a).

	α_s-CN	β-CN	k-CN	α-LA	β-LG	SP	SE
SU	1.12^{A}	0.79^{A}	0.27	0.16	0.38	0.29^{B}	0.08
SP	1.36^{B}	0.97^{B}	0.25	0.17	0.38	0.18^{A}	0.10

A,B Means within a column with different superscript letters differ (P<0.01).
CN = casein.
LA = lactalbumin.
LG = lactoglobulin.
SP = serum proteins.
SE: standard error of the model.

With regard to other dairy ruminants, Sevi et al. (2001) documented that the exposure of dairy sheep to solar radiation under HAT causes a lower yield of casein.

Health

It is generally stated that HS can be associated with a higher incidence of health problems (Martin et al., 1975; Webster et al., 1983; Silanikove, 2000; Kadzere et al., 2002; Lopes-Gatius et al., 2002).

First of all, HAT can modify the incidence of some parasitic diseases by indirect mechanisms because vectors and/or pathogens in some cases thrive better in hot and humid environment (Silanikove, 2000; Kadzere et al., 2002).

Secondly, high environmental temperatures, and heat waves in particular, can result in death losses for livestock (Hahn et al., 2002).

Furthermore, metabolic changes (DuBois & Williams, 1980; Pavlicek et al., 1989; Lacetera et al., 1996), pro-oxidant antioxidant balance (Harmon et al., 1997; Trout et al., 1998; Bernabucci et al., 2002b), and changes of the immune functions (Soper et al. 1978; Kelley et al. 1982; Elvinger et al. 1991; Kamwanja et al. 1994; Nardone et al., 1997; Lacetera et al., 2002) may represent examples of HS-related phenomena, which can play a role in modifying health of ruminants.

Metabolic status

Reduction of feed intake and other physiological responses to HAT (increase of maintenance requirements, panting, sweating, etc.) determine, in dairy cows and sheep, significant variations of biochemical indices of energy, protein and mineral metabolism and liver function (Ronchi et al., 1995), which can lead to metabolic disorders.
Pavlicek et al. (1989) reported that HS increases significantly the incidence of ketosis in dairy cows. Accordingly, the exposure of early lactating cows to HAT is responsible for hypoglycaemia, high values of non esterified fatty acids (NEFA) and β-hydroxy butyrate indicating energy deficit, massive lipomobilization and sub-clinical ketosis (Lacetera et al., 1996). Accordingly, the exposure of sheep to solar radiation under HAT caused decrease of plasma glucose (Bertoni et al., 1991) or increase of plasma NEFA (Sevi et al., 1991).
Exposure of dairy cows to HAT is also responsible for significant reduction of the synthetic ability of the liver, as testified by the reduction of plasma albumin and cholesterol, and for a certain degree of hepatobiliary disorders (Ronchi et al., 1999).
Panting during HS is responsible for loss of carbon dioxide (CO_2) and rise of plasma pH, which can lead to respiratory alkalosis both in dairy cows and sheep (Sanchez et al., 1994; Bernabucci et al., unpublished). Either in cows or sheep, losses of CO_2 (panting), potassium (sweating) and sodium (urine) and reduction of tubular acid (chlorine) secretion are responsible for reduction of cation-anion balance (sodium + potassium - chlorine) (West et al., 1992; Ronchi et al., 1997; Sevi et al., 2001).
Finally, DuBois & Williams (1980) reported a higher incidence of retained placenta in dairy cows calving in summer.

Prooxidant-antioxidant balance

Oxidative stress resulting from increased production of free radicals and reactive oxygen species and/or decrease in antioxidant defence, leads to damage of biological macromolecules and disruption of normal metabolism and physiology (Trevisan et al., 2001). When reactive forms of oxygen are produced faster than they can be safely neutralised by antioxidant mechanisms, oxidative stress results (Sies, 1991). These conditions can contribute and/or lead to the onset of health problems in cattle (Miller et al., 1993).
Harmon et al. (1997) described reduction of antioxidant activity of plasma in heat stressed mid-lactating cows. Trout et al., 1998 reported no effects of short exposure to HAT on concentration of lipid soluble antioxidants (α-tocopherol, β-carotene, retinol and retinyl palmitate) and on concentration of MDA in muscle. Calamari et al. (1999) found reduction of plasma lipid soluble antioxidants (vitamin E and β-carotene), and increase of plasma thiobarbituric acid reactive substances (TBARs) in heat stressed and mid-lactating cows.
In a recent field study (Bernabucci et al., 2002b) we found that moderate HS did not modify plasma markers of the oxidative status in transition cows. In contrast, in the same study we described differences in the oxidative status of summer and spring cows by considering erythrocyte markers (Table 2). In particular, erythrocytes from summer cows had higher superoxide dismutase (SOD) and glutathione peroxidase (GSH-Px-E) activities, intracellular thiol contents (SH) and TBARs.

Table 2. Least square means ± SE of the means of erythrocyte lipid peroxidation-end products (TBARS), superoxide dismutase activity (SOD), glutathione peroxidase (GSH-Px-E) activity, and intracellular thiols (SH) of summer (SU) and spring (SP) cows during the transition period (Bernabucci et al., 2002b).

Days from calving		TBARS nmol/ml	SOD U/ml	GSH-Px-E U/ml PCV[1]	SH µmol/ml PCV
-21	SU	8.3 ± 0.4[B]	176.4 ± 19.8	65.7 ± 3.9[b]	210.3 ± 56.3[b]
	SP	7.5 ± 0.4[A]	141.4 ± 18.8	46.4 ± 3.7[a]	119.0 ± 53.4[a]
-3	SU	9.1 ± 0.4[b]	194.3 ± 20.3[b]	69.6 ± 4.0	307.9 ± 57.7[B]
	SP	7.5 ± 0.4[a]	140.5 ± 20.0[a]	62.3 ± 4.0	161.5 ± 57.0[A]
1	SU	10.2 ± 0.4[B]	215.3 ± 21.3[b]	59.4 ± 4.2	282.8 ± 60.6[B]
	SP	7.0 ± 0.4[A]	179.0 ± 18.8[a]	56.0 ± 3.7	153.8 ± 53.4[A]
15	SU	8.6 ± 0.4	192.8 ± 21.3[b]	62.9 ± 3.9	295.1 ± 60.6[B]
	SP	8.1 ± 0.4	143.0 ± 18.8[a]	56.9 ± 3.7	116.2 ± 53.4[A]
35	SU	8.8 ± 0.4[b]	153.0 ± 19.8[b]	56.6 ± 3.9	289.3 ± 56.3[b]
	SP	7.6 ± 0.4[a]	172.8 ± 20.0[a]	52.2 ± 4.0	139.5 ± 57.0a

[1]PCV = Packed cells volume.
a,bMean within column with different superscript within parameter differ ($P<0.05$).
A,BMean within column with different superscript within parameter differ ($P<0.01$).

The first conclusions from that study were that moderate HS can cause oxidative stress in transition dairy cows, and that erythrocytes and not plasma markers may be an appropriate model to study the oxidative status of moderately heat stressed transition dairy cows. The high content of polyunsaturated fatty acid in erythrocyte membranes, and their continuous exposure to high concentration of oxygen and iron in haemoglobin are the factors that make erythrocytes very sensitive to the oxidative injury (Clemens & Waller, 1987) and an appropriate model to study oxidative stress (Alicigüzel et al., 2001).
Secondly, we speculated that the co-ordinate increase of erythrocyte SOD, GSH-Px-E, and SH would represent an indirect compensatory response of cells to increased oxidant challenge during HS (Yu, 1994). On the other hand, the increment in erythrocyte TBARs indicates that the balance between the oxidants and the antioxidants was in favour of the former. The hypothesis done was that the increased risk of oxidation for the erythrocytes would be represented by the higher $^{\bullet}O_2^-$ generation, which in turn would be due to the increase of oxygen pressure of blood due to the increased respiratory rate taking place during HS.
In sheep, the exposure to HAT causes increase of plasma ROMs and decrease of plasma SHp, which confirm that HS can cause alterations of the oxidative status (Bernabucci et al., unpublished).

Immune functions

It has been reported that the effects of HAT on resistance to infectious diseases or immune responsiveness of homeothermic animals depend on several variables, such as species and breed, duration of the exposure, severity of the stress, or type of the immune response taken into consideration (Kelley 1982).

A higher susceptibility to infections has been reported for cows suffering from HS (Webster, 1983), and a series of studies has been carried out to assess the relationships between HS and immune functions of bovines (Soper et al. 1978; Kelley et al. 1982a, b; Elvinger et al. 1991; Kamwanja et al. 1994; Lacetera et al., 2002a; Lacetera et al., unpublished). However, probably due to marked differences in the experimental conditions, results of those studies are conflicting. Soper and co-workers (1978) described a summer increase of proliferation in mitogen-stimulated lymphocytes of Holstein dairy cows. Working with calves, Kelley et al. (1982a) concluded that HS is responsible for alterations of the immune response, and that the HS-induced changes in immune events depend on the type of the immune response, and the length of time that calves are exposed to the stressor. In another study, still undertaken with calves, the same authors (Kelley et al. 1982b) found that HS had no direct effects on proliferation of mitogens-stimulated peripheral blood mononuclear cells (PBMCs). Furthermore, two in vitro studies demonstrated that exposure of bovine lymphocytes to short and severe heat shock reduced responsiveness to mitogens or decreased the number of viable cells (Elvinger et al. 1991; Kamwanja et al. 1994). Recently, we reported that moderate HS did not affect significantly proliferation of mitogens-stimulated PBMCs (Lacetera et al., 2002). Furthermore, in another study (unpublished) we also observed that HS would mask the impairment of the immune response reported for cows approaching to calving.

Sevi et al. (2001) reported that dairy sheep exposed to solar radiation under HAT showed a lower response to the intradermal injection of phytohemagglutinin that represents an indication of depressed cell-mediated immune response.

Finally, in a recent climatic chamber experiment carried out with dairy goats (unpublished) we found that the exposure to HAT increased proliferation of mitogen-stimulated PBMCs (Figure 2). The higher reactivity of PBMCs isolated from heat stressed ruminants might be due to the heat stress related changes of endocrine status (Johnson 1987; Ronchi et al., 2001). In particular, chronic heat stress is associated either with decline of immunodepressant hormones, namely glycocorticoids (Kelley, 1982), or with increase of prolactin, which in other species acts as strong stimulator of lymphocyte proliferation (Buckley, 2000).

Conflicting results have also been reported on the relationships between season or HS and colostral content of immunoglobulins (Ig) in dairy cows (Kruse 1970; Shearer et al. 1992; Nardone et al. 1997; Lacetera 1998; Lacetera et al., 2002). Kruse (1970) and Shearer et al. (1992) reported respectively that total Ig concentration in summer colostrum did not differ or was higher when compared to that recorded during other seasons. In a study carried out in climatic chambers, Nardone et al. (1997) found that THI values capable of determining severe HS were associated with significant reductions of colostral IgG and IgA in primiparous dairy cows. Authors explained their results by demonstrating a reduced passage of IgG from bloodstream to the udder, and hypothesising an impairment of the immune reactivity of the mammary gland plasmacytes to synthesise IgA. Finally, in the study already cited above (Lacetera et al., 2002), it has been reported that moderate HS does not modify the protective value of cows colostrum.

Different studies undertaken either under field conditions or controlled environment, documented higher mortality rate or impairment of passive immunisation in calves born during summer (Martin et al. 1975; Stott 1980; Donovan et al. 1986; Nardone et al., 1994; Lacetera 1998). Martin et al. (1975) documented a higher mortality rate of calves born during summer. Stott (1980) demonstrated an impairment of Ig absorption in calves born in hot environments. Donovan et al. (1986) found lower plasma Ig in summer post-colostral calves. Nardone et al. (1994) reported that calves born in hot environment and fed colostrum produced by dams exposed to heat during late pregnancy and early post-partum period showed, if compared to counterparts born under thermal comfort conditions, slower increase of plasma Ig and lower levels of Ig at the end of the absorptive period. Finally, in contrast with these results in a recent field study we observed that moderate HS in dairy cows is not associated with changes in passive immunisation of their offspring (Lacetera et al., 2002).

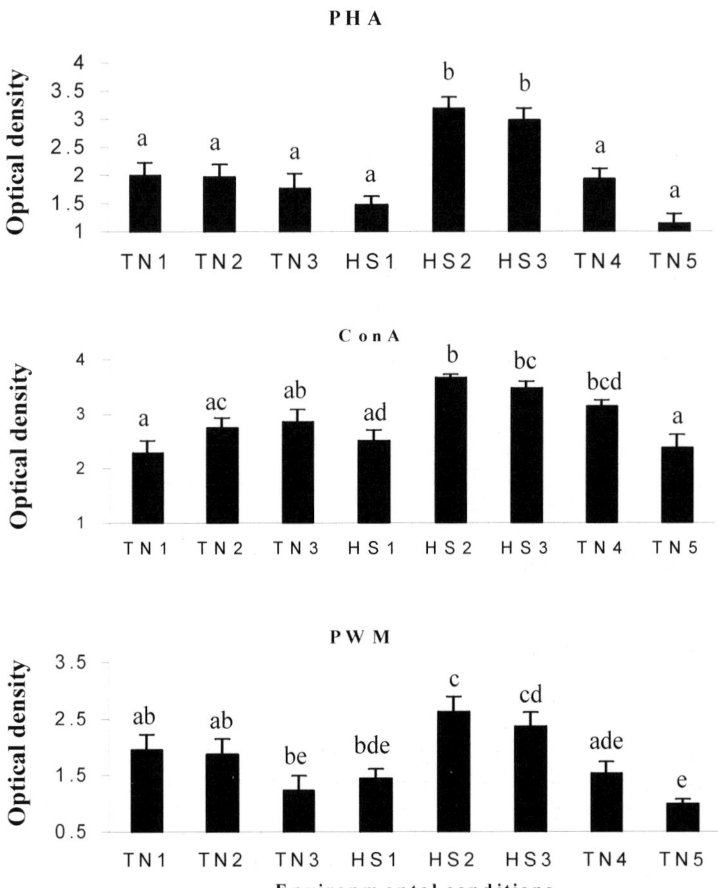

Figure 2. Least square means ± SE of the means of the DNA synthesis in peripheral blood mononuclear cells isolated from goats exposed to thermoneutral (TN) or heat stress conditions (HS) for 5 and 3 weeks, respectively, and stimulated with phytohemagglutinin (PHA), concanavalin A (ConA) and pokeweed mitogen (PWM). Columns with different letters differ significantly ($P<0.01$).

Conclusions

This paper pointed out that most of the literature referred to the effects of HS on physiology and productivity of intensively managed dairy ruminants is referred to dairy cows, and that the interest of researchers in this field is still high after approximately half century from first qualified demonstrations (Brody, 1956). To us, one of the reasons of such longevity stays probably in the continuous increase of the yielding capacity of dairy ruminants, which made progressively more marked the negative effects of HAT.

Quality of colostrum and milk produced from heat stressed dairy ruminants authorises to indicate that colostrum and milk produced and consumed during hot seasons is not equivalent to those yielded and consumed in other periods of the year.
With regard to the effects of HAT on health of dairy ruminants, HS can be responsible for metabolic and/or oxidative stress, which can contribute to the onset of diseases.
Results on the effects of HS on the immune response of dairy ruminants are dramatically conflicting, and in practice the only aspects of the immunity studied up to now have been the lymphocyte response to mitogens, protective value of cows colostrum and passive immunisation of calves. Further studies are encouraged to verify the effects of HS in dairy ruminants on other crucial aspects of the immunoresponsiveness (i.e., antibody and cytokine secretions), or on the effective resistance of heat stressed dairy ruminants to infections. Finally, also of interest would seem further epidemiological studies in dairy ruminants assessing the effective risk of infections through the year in order to establish whether HAT have to be associated with changes in the incidence of infections.

Acknowledgements

Research on the effects of heat stress on the immune responses of goats have been funded by MIUR (FIRB project).

References

Aliciguzel Y., Ozdem S.N., Ozdem S.S., Karayalc U., Siedlak S.L., Perry G. & Shith M.A., 2001. Erythrocyte, plasma, and serum antioxidant activities in untreated toxic multinodular goiter patients. Free Radic. Biol. Med. 30: 665–670.

Ames D.R., Brink D.R. & Willms C.L., 1980. Adjusting protein in feedlot diets during thermal stress. J. Anim. Sci. 50: 1-6.

Armstrong D.V., 1994. Heat stress interaction with shade and cooling. J. Dairy Sci. 77: 2044-2050.

Baccari F., Johnson H.D. & Hahn G.L., 1983. Environmental heat effects on growth, plasma T3, and postheat compensatory effects on holstein calves. Proc. Soc. Exp. Biol. Med. 173: 312-318.

Barash H., Silanikove N., Shamay A. & Ezra E, 2001. Interrelationships among ambient temperature, day length, and milk yield in dairy cows under a Mediterrannean climate. J. Dairy Sci. 84 (10): 2314-2320.

Bernabucci U. & Calamari L., 1998. Effect of heat stress on bovine milk yield and composition, Zootec. Nutr. Anim. 24: 247–257.

Bernabucci U., Lacetera N., Ronchi B. & Nardone A., 2002a. Effects of the hot season on milk protein fractions in Holstein cows. Anim. Res. 51: 25–33.

Bernabucci U., Ronchi B., Lacetera N. & Nardone A., 2002b. Markers of oxidative status in plasma and erythrocytes of transition dairy cows during hot season. J. Dairy Sci. 85: 2173–2179.

Bertoni G., Bernabucci U. & Filippi Balestra G., 1991. Heat stress effects on some blood parameters of sheep. In: Proc. Symp. Animal husbandry in warm climates. EAAP Publ. NO. 55: 98-102.

Bianca W., 1965. Reviews of the progress of dairy science. Physiology. Cattle in hot environment. J. Dairy Sci. 32: 291-328.

Brody S., 1956. Climatic physiology of cattle. J. Dairy Sci. 39: 715- 725.

Buckley AR., 2001. Prolactin, a lymphocyte growth and survival factor. Lupus 10: 684-90.

Calamari L. & Mariani P., 1998. Effects of the hot environment conditions on the main milk cheesemaking properties. Zootec. Nutr. Anim. 24: 259–271.

Calamari L., Maianti M. G., Amendola F. & Lombardi G., 1999. On some aspects of the oxidative status and on antioxidants in blood of dairy cows during summer. In: Proc. XIII Congress Associazione Scientifica Produzioni Animali 449–451.

Catillo G., Macciotta N.P., Carretta A. & Cappio-Borlino A., 2002. Effects of age and calving season on lactation curves of milk production traits in Italian water buffaloes. J. Dairy Sci. 85 (5): 1298-1306.

Clemens M. C. & Waller H.D., 1987. Lipid peroxidation in erythrocytes. Chem. Phys. Lipids. 45: 251–268.

Collier R.J., Doelger S.G., Head H.H., Thatcher W.W. & Wilcox C.J., 1982. Effects of heat stress during pregnancy on maternal hormone concentrations, calf birth weight and postpartum milk yield of holstein cows. J. Anim. Sci. 54: 309-319.

DuBois P.R. & Williams D.J., 1980. Increased incidence of retained placenta associated with heat in dairy cows. Theriogenology 13: 115-121.

Elvinger F., Hansen P.J. & Natzke R.P., 1991. Modulation of function of bovine polimorphonuclear leukocytes and lymphocytes by high temperature *in vitro* and *in vivo*. Am. J. Vet. Res. 52: 1692-1698

Forar F.L., Kincaid R.L., Preston R.L. & Hillers J.K., 1982. Variation of inorganic phosphorus in blood, plasma and milk of lactating cows, J. Dairy Sci. 65: 760–763.

Gallacier J.P., Barbier J.P. & Kuzdzal-Savoie S., 1974. Seasonal changes of relative proportion of milk fatty acids in d'Ille-et-Vilaine region. Le Lait 533-534: 117-138.

Gilad E., Meidan R., Berman A., Graber Y & Wolfenson D., 1993 Effect of heat stress on tonic and GnRH-induced gonadotrophin secretion in relation to concentration of oestradiol in plasma of cyclic cows. J. Reprod. Fert., 99: 315-321.

Gwazdauskas F.C., 1985. Effects of climate on reproduction in cattle. J. Dairy Sci., 68: 1568-1578.

Hahn G.L., Mader T.L., Harrington J.A., Nienaber J.A. & Frank K.L., 2002. Living with climatic variability and potential global change: climatological analyses of impacts on livestock performance. In: Proc. 15th Conf. Biometeorol. Aerobiol. 45-49.

Harmon, R.J., Lu M., Trammel D.S. & Smith B.A., 1997. Influence of heat stress and calving on antioxidant activity in bovine blood. J. Dairy Sci. 80 (Suppl. 1): 264.

Hermansen J.E., Ostersen S., Justesen N.C. & Aaes O., 1999. Effects of dietary protein supply on caseins, whey proteins, proteolysis and renneting properties in milk from cows grazing clover or N-fertilized grass, J. Dairy Res. 66: 193–205.

Johnson H.D., Ragsdale A.C., Berry I.L. & Shanklin M.D., 1962. Effects of various temperature-humidity combinations on milk production of Holstein cattle. Mo. Agric. Exp. Station Res. Bull. 791.

Johsnon H.D., 1987. Bioclimate effects on growth, reproduction and milk production. In: Bioclimatology and Adaptation of Livestock, Elsevier Sci. Publ., B.V., Amsterdam, The Netherlands, 35-57.

Johnson H.D., Shanklin M.D. & Hahn L., 1988a. Productive adaptability of Holstein cows to environmental heat. Mo. Agric. Exp. Station Res. Bull. 1060.

Johnson H.D., Katti P.S., LeRoy H.G. & Shanklin M.D., 1988b. Short term heat acclimation effects on hormonal profile of lactating cows. Mo. Agric. Exp. Station Res. Bull. 1061.

Kadzere C.T., Murphy M.R., Silanikove N. & Maltz E., 2002. Heat stress in lactating dairy cows: a review. Livest. Prod. Sci. 77: 59-91.

Kamwanja L.A., Chase Jr. C.C., Gutierrez J.A., Guerriero V.J., Olson T.A., Hammond A.C. & Hansen P.J., 1994. Responses of bovine lymphocytes to heat shock as modified by breed and antioxidant status. J. Anim. Sci. 72: 438-444.

Kelley K.W., 1982. Immunobiology of domestic animals as affected by hot and cold weather. In. Proc. 2nd International Livestock Environment Symposium. ASAE Publ. 3–82. ASAE, St. Joseph, Mich. 470–483

Kelley K.W., Greenfield R.E., Evermann J.F., Parish S.M. & Perryman L.E., 1982a. Delayed-type hypersensitivity, contact sensitivity, and phytohemagglutinin skin-test responses of heat- and cold-stressed calves. Am. J. Vet. Res. 43: 775-779.

Kelley K.W., Osborne C.A., Evermann J.F., Parish S.M. & Gaskins C.T., 1982b. Effects of chronic heat and cold stressors on plasma immunoglobulin and mitogen-induced blastogenesis in calves. J. Dairy Sci. 65: 1514-1528.

Kume S., Takahashi S., Kurihara M. & Aii T., 1989. The effects of a hot environment on the major mineral content in milk. Japanese J. Zootech. Sci. 60: 341-345.

Lacetera N., Ronchi B., Bernabucci U. & Nardone A., 1994. Influence of heat stress on some biometric parameters and on body condition score in female Holstein calves. Rivista Agric. Subtrop. e Trop. 88 (1): 81-89.

Lacetera N., Bernabucci U., Ronchi B. & Nardone A., 1996. Body condition score, metabolic *status* and milk production of early lactating dairy cows exposed to warm environment. Rivista Agric. Subtrop. e Trop. 90 (1): 43-55.

Lacetera N., 1998. Influence of high air temperatures on colostrum composition of dairy cows and passive immunization of calves. Zootec. Nutr. Anim. 6: 239-246.

Lacetera N., Bernabucci U., Ronchi B., Scalia D. & Nardone A., 2002. Moderate summer heat stress does not modify immunological parameters of Holstein dairy cows. Int. J. Biometeorol. 46: 33-37.

Linvil D.E. & Pardue F.E., 1992. Heat stress and milk production in South Carolina coastal plains. J. Dairy Sci. 75: 2598-2604.

Lopes-Gatius F., Santolaria P., Yaniz J., Fenech M. & Lopez-Bejar M., 2002. Risk factors for postpartum ovarian cysts and their spontaneous recovery or persistence in lactating dairy cows. Theriogenology 58 (8): 1623-1632.

Mackle T.R., Bryant A.M., Petch S.F., Hill J.P. & Auldist M.J., 1999. Nutritional influences on the composition of milk from cows of different protein phenotypes in New Zealand. J. Dairy Sci. 82: 172–180.

Mariani P., Zanzucchi G., Blanco P. & Masoni M., 1993. Variazioni stagionali del contenuto in fosforo del latte di massa di singoli allevamenti. L'Industria del Latte 29: 39-53.

Mariani P., Summer A., Maffezzoli F. & Znanzucchi G., 1995. Variazioni stagionali della resa del latte in formaggio Grana Padano. Annali Facoltà MedicinaVeterinaria Parma. 15: 159–166.

Martin S.W., Schwabe C.W. & Franti C.E., 1975. Dairy calf mortality rate: characteristics of calf mortality rates in Tulare County. California. Am. J. Vet. Res. 36: 1099–1104.

McDowell R.E., Moody E.G., Van Soest P.J., Lehmann R.P. & Ford G.L., 1969. Effect of heat stress on energy and water utilization of lactating cows. J. Dairy Sci. 52: 188-194.

Mercier J.C. & Gaye P., 1983. Milk protein synthesis. In: Mepham T.B. (editor), Biochemistry of Lactation, Elsevier Sci. Publ., B.V., Amsterdam, The Netherlands,177–230.

Miller J.K., Brzezinska-Slebodzinska E. & Madsen F.C., 1993. Oxidative stress, antioxidants, and animal function. J. Dairy Sci. 76: 2812–2823.

Moe P.W., Tyrrell H.F. & Flatt W.P., 1971. Energetics of body tissue mobilisation. J. Dairy Sci. 54: 548-553.

Nardone A., Lacetera N., Ronchi B. & Bernabucci U., 1992. Effetti dello stress termico sulla produzione di latte e sui consumi alimentari di vacche Frisone. Prod. Anim. 5: 1-15.

Nardone A., Lacetera N., Ronchi B. & Bernabucci U., 1993. Consumo di alimento ed accrescimento in vitelle di razza Frisona esposte a condizioni di *stress* termico. In: Proc. X° Congress Associazione Scientifica Produzioni Animali 155-159.

Nardone A., Lacetera N.G., Ronchi B. & Bernabucci U., 1994. Effect of heat stress in primiparous dairy cows on colostrum composition and on passive immunisation of calves. In: Proc. 45th Annual Meeting E.A.A.P. 193.

Nardone A., Lacetera N., Bernabucci U. & Ronchi B., 1997. Composition of colostrum from dairy heifers exposed to high air temperatures during late pregnancy and the early postpartum period. J. Dairy Sci. 80 (5): 838-844.

NRC, 1981. Effects of environment on nutrient requirements of domestic animals. National Academy Press, Washington D.C. 152.

Ozimek L. & Kennelly J., 1994. The effect of seasonal and regional variation in milk composition on potential cheese yield. FIL-IDF Bull. No. 9402: 95–100.

Palmquist D.L., Beaulieu A.D. & Barbano D.M., 1993 Feed and animal factors influencing milk fat composition. J. Dairy Sci. 76: 1753-1771.

Paula-Lopes F.F., Chase C.C., Al-Katanani Y.M., Kriniger III C.E., Rivera R.M., Tekin S., Majewski A.C., Ocon O.M., Olson T.A. & Hansen P.J., 2003. Genetic divergence in cellular resistance to heat shock in cattle: differences between breeds developed in temperate versus hot climates in responses of preimplantation embryos, reproductive tract tissues and lymphocytes to increased culture temperatures. Reprod. 125: 285-294.

Pavlicek A., Misljenovic Z. & Misic M., 1989. Uticaj visokih ljetnjih temperatura na proizvodnju mlijeka, zdravlje krava I plodnost. Vet. Glasnik 43: 397-400.

Piva G., Fusconi G., Prandini A. & Capri E., 1993. Composizione acidica del grasso del latte: fattori di variabilità in aziende dell'area padana. Sci. Tecn. Lattiero-Casearia 44: 309-323.

Ravagnolo O. & Misztal I., 2002. Effect of Heat Stress on Nonreturn Rate in Holsteins: Fixed-Model Analyses. J. Dairy Sci. 85: 3101–3106.

Rodtian P, King G, Subrod S & Pongpiachan P., 1996. Oestrous behaviour of Holstein cows during cooler and hotter tropical seasons. Anim. Reprod. Sci. 45 (1-2): 47-58.

Ronchi B., Bernabucci U., Lacetera N. & Nardone A. 1995. Milk fatty acid composition in cows exposed to hot environment. In: Proc. XI° Congress Associazione Scientifica Produzione Animale 353-354.

Ronchi B., Bernabucci U., Lacetera N., Nardone A., 1997. Effetti dello stress termico sullo stato metabolico-nutrizionale di vacche Frisone in lattazione. Zootec. Nutr. Anim. 23: 3-15.

Ronchi B., Bernabucci U., Lacetera N., Verini Supplizi A. & Nardone A. 1999. Distinct and common effects of heat stress and restricted feeding on metabolic status of holstein heifers. Zootec. Nutr. Anim. 1: 11-20.

Ronchi B., Stradaioli G., Verini Supplizi A., Bernabucci U., Lacetera N., Accorsi P.A., Nardone A. & Seren E., 2001. Influence of heat stress or feed restriction on plasma progesterone, oestradiol-17β, LH, FSH, prolactin and cortisol in Holstein heifers. Livest. Prod. Sci. 68 (2-3): 231-241.

Sanchez W.K., McGuire M.A. & Beede D.K., 1994. Macromineral nutrition by heat stress interactions in dairy cattle: review and original research. J. Dairy Sci. 77: 2051-2079.

Sano H., Ambo K. & Tsuda T., 1985. Blood glucose kinetics in whole body and mammary gland of lactating goats exposed to heat. J. Dairy Sci. 68 (10): 2557-2564.

Schmidt D.G., 1980. Colloidal aspects of casein. Neth. Milk Dairy J. 34: 42–64.

Sevi A., Annichiarico G., Albenzio M., Taibi L., Muscio A. & Dell'Aquila S., 2001. Effects of solar radiation and feeding time on behavior, immune response and production of lactating ewes under high ambient temperature. J. Dairy Sci., 84: 629-640.

Sevi A., Rotunno T., Di Caterina R. & Muscio A., 2002. Fatty acid composition of ewe milk as affected by solar radiation and high ambient temperature. J. Dairy Res. 69: 181-194.

Sies, H., 1991. Oxidative Stress: Oxidants and Antioxidants. Academic Press, San Diego, CA, 650.

Silanikove N., 2000. Effects of heat stress on the welfare of extensively managed domestic ruminants. Livest. Prod. Sci. 67: 1-18.

Smith G.H., Grabtree B. & Smith R.A., 1983. Energy metabolism in the mammary gland. In: Biochemistry of Lactation. Mepham T.B. (editor) Elsevier Sci. Publ., B.V., Amsterdam, The Netherlands, 121-140.

Soper F., Muscoplat C.C. & Johnson D.W., 1978. In vitro stimulation of bovine peripheral blood lymphocytes: analysis of variation of lymphocyte blastogenic response in normal dairy cattle. Am. J. Vet. Res. 39: 1039–1042

Trevisan, M., Browne R., Ram M., Muti P., Freudenheim J., Carosella A.N. & Armstrong. D., 2001. Correlates of markers of oxidative status in the general population. Am. J. Epidemiol. 154: 348–356.

Trout J. P., McDowell L. R. & Hansen P. J., 1998. Characteristics of the estrous cycle and antioxidant status of lactating Holstein cows exposed to heat stress. J. Dairy Sci. 81: 1244–1250.

Urech E. & Puhan Z., 1992. Yield of cheese and butter in Emmental cheese factories: a case of study, Schweiz. Milchw. Forsch. 21: 30–37.

Webster A.J.F., 1983. Environmental stress and the physiology, performance and health of ruminants. J. Anim. Sci. 57: 1584- 1593.

Webster A.J.F., 1987. Understanding the dairy cow. BSP Professional Books, Oxford, England, 357.

West J.W., Haydon K.D., Mullinix B.G. & Sandifer T.G., 1992. Dietary cation-anion balance and cation source effects on production and acid.base status of heat-stressed cows. J. Dairy Sci. 75: 2776-2786.

West J.W., Mullinix B.G. & Bernard J.K., 2003. Effects of hot, humid weather on milk temperature, dry matter intake and milk yield of lactating dairy cows. J. Dairy Sci. 86: 232-242.

Wilson S.J., Marion R.S., Spain J.N., Spiers D.E., Keisler D.H. & Lucy M.C., 1998. Effects of controlled heat stress on ovarian function of dairy cattle: 1. Lactating cows. J. Dairy Sci. 81: 2124-2131.

Wise M.E., Rodriguez R.E., Armstrong D.V., Huber J.T., Weirsma F. & Hunter R., 1988. Fertility and hormonal responses to temporary relief of heat stress in lactating dairy cows. Theriogenology 29: 1027-1035.

Wolfenson D., Luft O., Berman A. & Meidan R., 1993. Effects of season , incubation temperature and cell age on progesterone and prostaglandin $F_{2\alpha}$ production in bovine luteal cells. Anim. Reprod. Sci. 32: 27-40.

Wolfenson D., Roth Z. & Meidan R., 2000. Impaired reproduction in heat-stressed cattle: basic and applied aspects. Anim. Reprod. Sci. 60-61: 535-547.

Yousef M.K., 1987. Principles of Bioclimatology. In: Bioclimatology and Adaptation of Livestock, Elsevier Sci. Publ., B.V., Amsterdam, The Netherlands, 17-31.

Yu B.P., 1994. Cellular defenses against damage from reactive oxygen species. Physiol. Rev. 74: 139-162.

Novel approaches for the alleviation of climatic stress in farm animals

R.J. Collier, C. Coppola & A. Wolfgram

Department of Animal Sciences, University of Arizona, 85721 Tucson, Arizona, USA, rcollier@ag.arizona.edu

Summary

New management tools have become available to assist in identifying and evaluating stress in domestic animals. One example is infrared thermometry, which permits the evaluation of skin temperature of livestock to determine their cooling needs. Studies conducted at the University of Arizona indicate that surface temperatures above 35^{0}C will result in elevated respiration rates and rectal temperatures in cattle. Development of gene expression microarrays will soon accelerate the identification of genes associated with resistance or sensitivity to stressors. However, there is need to differentiate between gene expression related to acclimation as opposed to those associated with adaptation. Review of literature indicates variability among animals in resistance to cold stress is greater than variability across animals in resistance to heat stress. Estimates of genotype by environment interactions with respect to resistance to thermal stress have been low or non-existent when comparisons are made within the same environments. Comparisons within the same cattle breeds across several countries and environments have yielded larger estimates. Increase in milk yield of lactating dairy cows and resulting increase in heat production over the last half century requires reevaluation of the relationship between milk yield and sensitivity to thermal stress. Thermal preconditioning to induce epigenetic heat adaptation has been demonstrated in poultry but has not yet been demonstrated in domestic mammals. Mouse lines divergently selected for heat loss had higher hypothalamic expression of oxytocin and tissue inhibitor of metalloproteinase 2 genes. Studies on cell cultures and whole organisms have identified genes associated with heat shock and other stress proteins as being related to thermo-resistance. The variability in promoter and coding regions of these genes is also connected to thermo-resistance and environmental conditions surrounding animals. However, over-expression of heat shock proteins as an approach to confer heat resistance may have deleterious effects on animal health including increased incidence of cancer. Induced acclimation through hormonal treatment of animals may offer a valuable tool in understanding the coordinated expression of many genes required to confer thermal resistance in domestic livestock.

Keywords: thermal stress, acclimation, adaptation, genomics

Introduction

Heat acclimation is a long-term developmental process that increases the dynamic body temperature regulatory range by lowering the body temperature threshold for activation of heat dissipation effectors and increasing the capacity of those effectors (Horowitz, 2001). It is a within lifetime event as opposed to adaptation, an evolutionary process which increases the fitness of a given species for climatic changes present in its ecological niche. Acclimatory changes are generally lost if the stress disappears which has led some to assume there is no genetic basis. Thus, the genetic component of acclimation if it exists is not known. Intriguing however, is the fact that in some species such as poultry the exposure of chicks to high environmental heat during embryonic development results in permanent changes in responses to heat stress in adult animals, (Moraes et al., 2003). Another issue not well understood is whether the genes associated with acclimation are also those associated with adaptation to thermal stress. Generally, as animals acclimatize to environmental stressors they reduce or divert metabolizable energy from production to balance heat gain and loss (Lemerle & Goddard, 1986, Keister et al., 2002). Thus, it has generally been faster and easier to obtain production increases by altering the environment around animals. However, evaluating cooling needs of animals is usually only estimated using temperature-humidity (THI) indices. As stated by Neinaber et al.,1999, "producers require the means to recognize stress responses and take appropriate actions." A recent development is the ability to monitor thermal status of animals directly using infrared thermography and or radiotelemetry (Lefcourt & Goddard, 1986, McVicker et al., 2002, Wolfgram et al., 2003) to determine cooling requirements. One objective of this paper is to provide evidence that infrared thermography is a reliable and low cost tool for producers to evaluate cooling needs. An additional and longer-term approach is to identify genes associated with acclimation of domestic animals to thermal stress. Identification of genes associated with thermal resistance may permit identification of markers that can be used in accelerated breeding programs to increase resistance of animals to thermal stress. Rate of genetic progress in domestic animal breeding programs is driven by three factors; accuracy of markers for phenotypic traits, intensity of marker use and generation interval. Presently, genetic markers for phenotypic traits do not generally correspond to the coding regions for the genes of interest. They are located close to loci of traits of interest but lose their value over time due to genetic recombination. Ideally, genetic markers should identify the exact location of the gene of interest. Identifying these genes is of primary importance to any livestock improvement program. Therefore, a functional genomics approach to understanding the genetic mechanisms of heat stress, especially as related to production is warranted. Use of gene expression microarrays that permit evaluation of expression levels of thousands of genes at a time will rapidly increase knowledge of genes associated with resistance or sensitivity to environmental heat stress, such as those associated with increased evaporative heat loss capability. A second objective of this paper is to review available literature on candidate genes and research models to evaluate effects of environmental heat load on gene expression in cattle.

Materials and methods-infrared thermography

Two studies were carried out to evaluate relationship between ambient environmental conditions, cow surface temperatures and measures of heat stress. Infrared thermograms were captured of the udder (UIR) and side (SIR) using an infrared thermography camera (model eVS DTIS-500) manufactured by Emerge Vision[4]. Each image was taken using Look Up Table (LUT), color palette of 01 and a total viewable temperature range (RNG) of 07-11; this allowed for the broadest spectrum in depicted color. Any artifacts, dirt, manure etc., were removed prior to imaging. Surface temperatures of the udder (UG) and side (SG) were also measured using an infrared temperature gun manufactured by Raytek® (Raynger® MX™ model RayMX4PU).

Images from the camera were stored on a compact flash memory card (SanDisk®) and subsequently downloaded to a laptop computer for analysis using software from Emerge Vision, Diagnostic Thermal Imaging Software System 500. The software permitted analysis of temperatures within a specific area using an ellipse drawn on the desired area.

4 eMERGE Vision Systems, Inc. 10315 102nd Terrace Sebastian, Florida 32958

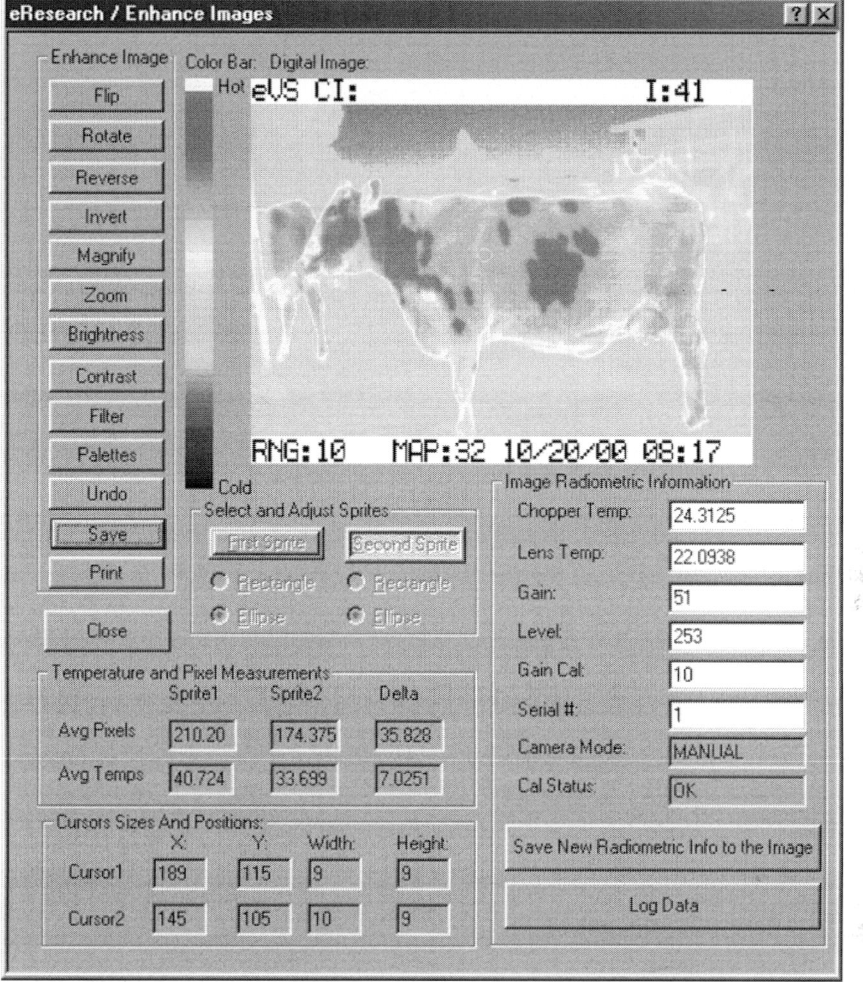

Figure 1. Infrared thermogram analysis of surface temperature in a Holstein cow.

As shown in Figure 1 The cow is standing in the open exposed to solar radiation. The surface temperature of the black hair coat is 40.7^{0}C while the surface temperature of the white hair coat is 33.7^0 C, a difference of 7°C.

The infrared camera and infrared gun were calibrated on a weekly basis using a copper globe painted flat black and a mercury thermometer. A hole was drilled in the top for water addition and insertion of a thermometer. The globe was filled with hot tap water and a mercury thermometer was inserted into the globe for temperature measurements for each calibration. At five-minute intervals a camera image, infrared gun reading and thermometer reading were taken for three calibration measurements.

Calibration data were analyzed (Statview, 1998) to establish the correlation between the infrared measurements and mercury thermometer measurements. Correlation values were compared between the infrared camera and black globe thermometer, the infrared gun and black globe thermometer and between the infrared camera and infrared gun. Both infrared devices were highly correlated (>93%) with the black globe thermometer and the two infrared devices had a high correlation (91%) to each other, Table 1.

Table 1. Correlation analysis from calibration data between Black Globe Thermometer and Infrared Camera, Black Globe Thermometer and Infrared Gun and between Infrared Camera and Infrared Gun.

Device	Correlation	N	P-Value	R^2
Black Globe Thermometer and Infrared Camera	0.937	41	<0.0001	0.879
Black Globe Thermometer and Infrared gun	0.95	41	<0.0001	0.903
Infrared Camera and Infrared Gun	0.913	41	<0.0001	0.834

The period for study one was June 19, 2000 to September 20, 2000. The average environment temperature for this period was 34°C with an average relative humidity of 32%. During the study period, the temperature humidity index (THI=0.72(W^0C = D^0C) + 40.6) ranged from 73.5 to 84.7.

Animals and data collection

Study 1

Four hundred Jersey cows were split into two treatment groups, cooled and non-cooled and 100 cows in each group were treated with bovine somatotropin (bST) (POSILAC®). Treatment groups were balanced for parity, milk yield and days postpartum. Cooled pens consisted of shade with fans and misters set to deliver approximately 21.2 m^3/m air and 14.3 L of water per hour per cow. Non-cooled pens consisted of shade only. Both groups were held in a similar cooled holding pen for approximately 30 minutes prior to milking each day. Once a week, measurements were taken between one and four pm on eight randomly chosen animals from each treatment group. Respiration rates per minute (visual observation) and surface temperatures of the udder and side were taken using an infrared thermography camera and an infrared temperature gun.

Study 2

Objective was to determine if infrared thermometry (gun) and thermography (camera) were more useful tools than temperature humidity index (THI) for assessing the thermal status of lactating dairy cattle and if so which infrared device is best to use. Three types of cooling structure for dairy cattle (shade with oscillating fans and misters, shade with Koral Kool™ coolers, and shade with stationary fans and misters) were compared for effectiveness in cooling lactating dairy cattle during warm summer months. The effectiveness of these systems were evaluated using an infrared temperature gun to measure side temperature, respiration rate of the cows when skin temperature was taken and milk yield of the animals. Data were collected thrice weekly from May through August 2001, from 116 lactating Holstein and Brown Swiss cows assigned to the three cooling regimes. Data from both studies were analyzed using a categorical model (SAS, 1996). An animal was classified as being in heat stress if respiration rate was greater than 85 respirations per minute. The models used to analyze the dependent variable heat stress included a separate model for each body temperature (SIR, UIR, SG or UG). Each model included the following independent variables: milk production the day prior to measurements, air temperature, stage of pregnancy, cooling treatment and bST treatment.

Results-infrared thermography

Study 1

All surface temperature measurements affected respiration rate ($P<0.007$) and therefore the classification of heat stress (RR>85 breaths/minute).The following variables also influenced respiration rate: temperature humidity index, bovine somatotropin treatment and cooling treatment ($P<0.04$) Milk production the day preceding measurements and stage of pregnancy did not have an affect on respiration rate ($P>0.05$).

The results of the analysis of environmental and animal factors on surface temperature measurements are shown in Table 2. The mean square (MS) and probability is shown for each surface temperature measurement for each variable. The THI measurement was taken outside the shade structures and did not affect surface temperatures under the shade systems. However, cooling under the shades was highly significant for each of the temperature measures taken.

This suggests that surface temperature measurements, taken directly on animals provides more information on thermal status of the animals than THI measurements of ambient conditions. Stage of pregnancy affected surface temperatures on the side of the animal but not the udder surface temperature. The use of bST did not affect surface temperature of the animals but there was an interaction between bST and cooling for side surface temperature as measured by the infrared gun ($P<0.05$), but not the infrared camera.

Cooling lowered all average surface temperature measurements. Average side surface temperature for cooled animals was 34.3^0C vs. 36.7^0C in uncooled animals. In addition, advancing pregnancy was associated with decreasing side but not udder surface temperatures. Average side surface temperatures for 1st, 2nd and 3rd trimesters was 37.5, 36.1 and 32.3^0 C respectively. The cause of this decrease in side surface temperature is unknown but pregnancy clearly exerts large effects on side surface temperature in cattle. Milk yield the day surface temperatures were recorded did not affect surface temperatures in this study, (Table 2). Since higher milk yields are associated with higher levels of heat production the possibility existed that this might affect side surface temperature. However, this was not the case. Use of bST to increase milk yield was also not associated with an increase in body surface temperatures in this study.

Study 2

Surface temperature and respiration rate were significantly different among the three cooling strategies. Analysis of the data indicated that infrared gun temperatures were more highly correlated with respiration rate ($r=0.73$, $P<0.001$), (Figure 2) than was THI ($r=0.51$, $P<0.001$), (figure not shown).

The infrared gun and infrared camera were also used to measure side surface temperatures during 3 circadian data collection periods in June, July and August, 2001. During each of the 3 collection periods both infrared measurements and respiration rates were taken each hour over a 24-hour period. Respiration rates were recorded by visual counting of chest movements over 15 seconds and multiplying by 4. Measurements were taken at night with the aid of a flashlight.

Table 2. Factors affecting surface temperature measurements in cattle in a semiarid environment.

Variance Source	df	SIR		UIR		SG		UG	
		MS	P	MS	P	MS	P	MS	P
THI	1	0.7017	0.7039	57.518	<0.0001	4.4058	0.3762	2.558	0.4162
Milk-Pre	1	15.703	0.0737	4.86	0.1511	1.8651	0.5643	0.0171	0.947
BST	1	0.0556	0.9148	0.024	0.9193	8.4177	0.2221	1.500	0.9987
Cooling	1	286.15	<0.0001	190.1	<0.0001	94.483	<0.0001	212.92	<0.0001
Stage of preg	3	33.824	0.0002	2.602	0.3448	39.932	0.0002	4.455	0.3279
bST x cooling	1	3.1095	0.4241	0.0543	0.8789	21.06	0.0548	0.1708	0.8335

SIR - side temperature from infrared camera
UIR - udder temperature from infrared camera
SG - side temperature from infrared temperature gun
UG - udder temperature from infrared temperature gun
P<.05 highlighted in red

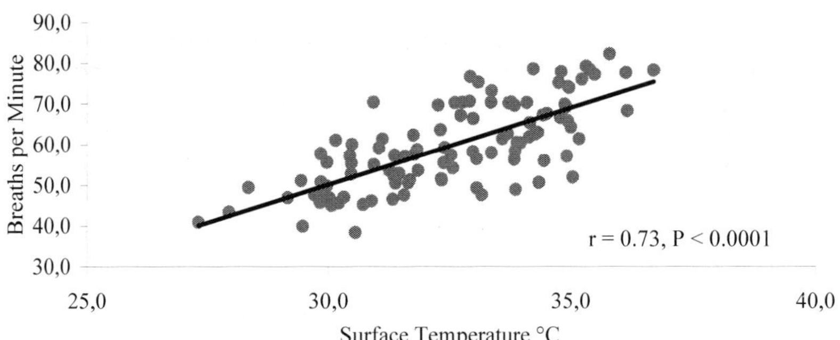

Figure 2. Relationship between infrared surface temperature and respiration rate in lactating Holstein cows.

Discussion

Infrared thermography

This study was designed to determine if heat stress had an affect on body surface temperature by using infrared temperature equipment. An animal was classified in heat stress if measured respiration rate was greater than 85 breaths per minute. Bovine dissipate heat and maintain thermal homeostasis through two mechanisms, sensible heat loss mechanisms (convection, conduction and radiation) which require a thermal gradient to operate and insensible or evaporative heat loss which works on a vapor/pressure gradient. Above the thermoneutral zone the only available route of heat loss for cattle is evaporative. Therefore, as ambient temperature increases respiration rates increase as well (Esmay, 1978, Ray et al., 1992).
This trend was shown in all treatment groups. When body surface temperature increased in both treatments (37.8°C vs. 35.5°C), cooled and non-cooled, respiration rates also increased. The respiration rate for non-cooled cows was significantly greater than cooled cows (102 breaths/min. vs. 80 breaths/min.).

It is generally accepted that ambient air temperature and solar radiation affect body temperature, and as observed by Lemerle & Goddard, 1986, body temperature affects respiration rate. As body temperature increases due to a lack of metabolic heat dissipation and high environmental heat load, respiration rates increase as well. As is shown in the present data, cooled cows are maintaining normal body temperature without increasing respiration rate because ambient conditions permit sensible heat loss mechanisms to operate.
From the two body temperatures measured, (side and udder), side temperature had the greatest association with respiration rate. This may be because the udder temperature is more affected by mammary metabolic activity than ambient conditions. From this data we conclude that it is possible to evaluate thermal status of unrestrained cattle using infrared thermography. Based on the relationship between skin surface temperature and respiration rate we conclude that a surface temperature below 35 °C is required to avoid increased core temperature and respiration rate. Furthermore, a simple infrared thermography gun that is available for less than $100 can be used to monitor cattle under group housing conditions. This permits the producer to evaluate cooling requirements regardless of weather conditions outside the housing system.

Acclimation and adaptation

The coordinated response of domestic animals to increased thermal heat load involves diversion of metabolizable energy to maintenance, reduced metabolism and heart rates, reduced production and lower body temperature, (Collier et al., 1982), (Beede & Collier, 1986). Animals are considered acclimated when body temperature returns to pre-stress levels, (Neinaber et al., 1999). Systemic, tissue, and cellular responses associated with acclimation are coordinated and require several days or weeks to occur and are therefore not homeostatic in nature, (Bligh, 1976). Some examples of these changes are shown in Table 3.

Table 3. Systemic components of acclimation to thermal stress.

Tissue	Species	Change	Reference
sweat gland	cattle	increased secretion	Manulu et al., 1991
hypothalamus	cattle	return to normal body rhythms	Nienaber et al., 1991
thyroid	chicken	decreased T_3	Moraes et al., 2003
thyroid	cattle	decreased T_3	Becker et al., 1990
muscle	rat	formation of myosin V3 (more efficient)	Horowitz et al., 1986
nerve	rat	increased sympathetic activity	Horowitz, 2001
adrenal	cattle	reduced corticoid secretion	Christian & Johnson. 1972
adrenal	cattle	reduced aldosterone secretion	Collier et al., 1982
pituitary	cattle	increased prolactin secretion	Thatcher, 1974

Furthermore, when the stress is removed these changes decay. This process of acclimation to a stress and subsequent reversion to the initial state are most noticeable as seasonal changes in animals exposed to the natural environment. Clearly, these changes involve reprogramming of gene expression. However, these changes are not permanent, do not involve change in the structure of genes and are not passed on to the next generation. However, it is not known if there is a genetic basis for differences within a given species in acclimation. When genotype x environment interactions are estimated in cattle there is considerable risk that the phenotypic response (acclimation) is confounded with the genotypic difference (adaptation).

Genotype x environment interactions

Evaluation of genetic basis for differences in acclimation and adaptation to thermal stress in domestic mammalian livestock populations has been limited by length of the lifecycle, cost of maintaining "lines" and small animal numbers. Estimates of genotype by environment interactions in cattle have been small when estimated within a single country and when examining data including temperature within the thermoneutral zone. There is some indication that estimates are larger when looking across several countries with corresponding larger ranges in environmental temperatures, (Ravagnolo et al., 2000, 2002), (Ravagnolo & Misztal, 2000), (Zwald et al., 2003). Ravagnolo & Misztal (2000) demonstrated that "for heat humidity indices below 72, heritability for milk was 0.17 and additive variance of heat tolerance was 0. For a heat humidity index of 86, the additive variance of heat tolerance was as high as for the general effect" Zwald et al., 2003 grouped thirteen management and environmental factors across 17 countries into quintiles based on herd averages for these variables. They found that genetic correlations for milk yield between quintiles were significantly less than for maximum monthly temperature indicating that this approach could be used to get better estimates of genotype x environment interactions within a given production environment. Additional work will need to be carried out to differentiate differences in acclimation versus adaptation in these traits.

Acclimation and homeorhesis

Homeorhesis is the coordination of metabolism to support a dominant physiological state (Bauman, 2000). The cellular and tissue changes associated with homeorhesis are remarkable similar to those found in acclimation, (Bligh, 1976). This strongly implies that acclimation is a homeorhetic process. If this is the case then homeorhetic regulators might be employed to assist in acclimation of animals to thermal stress. This was tested in a study conducted at the University of Missouri, (Becker et al., 1990) and (Manulu et al., 1991). These investigators hypothesized that bovine somatropin treatment of lactating dairy cows would increase milk yield and heat production. The increase in heat production during periods of high environmental temperature might then make the animals more susceptible to heat stress. Their data demonstrated that there was a large increase in milk yield and heat production of lactating dairy cows treated with bovine somatotropin. However, surprisingly, there was also a 36% increase in evaporative heat loss through increased sweating and respiration rate which allowed the cows to dissipate the increased heat load. Thus, the cows were hormonally acclimated permitting them to maintain normal body temperature. This may provide a useful model to evaluate which genes are turned on and off as animals adjust to higher heat production an increased heat loss via sweating and panting. Another hormone, which has been shown to increase during periods of thermal stress and may be associated with potassium turnover during thermal stress is prolactin, (Collier et al., 1982, Beede & Collier, 1986). Hormones which have been shown to coordinate metabolism such as thyroxine, prolactin and growth hormone may play a role in acclimation of domestic animals to environmental change.

Functional genomics

A major new set of tools in the study of genes associated with thermal sensitivity or resistance is the development of gene expression microarrays and real time polymerase chain reaction capabilities. These permit the simultaneous evaluation of the regulation of thousands of genes in response to environmental change. Biological models for this tool range from single cells to consomic lines of lab animals with single gene deletions to specific crosses of animals.

Combining use of these genetic models with single gene deletions and gene expression microarrays will rapidly increase knowledge of genes associated with tolerance or sensitivity to environmental heat stress.

Presently, few candidate genes for thermal tolerance have been identified, (Table 4). However, in the next few years gene expression arrays will identify a number of genes in a variety of species that are associated with responses to stressors.

Targets of potential genetic manipulation would include increased efficiency and capacity of thermal effectors and delayed onset of temperature threshold for thermal injury. For example, constitutive elevation of heat shock protein gene expression has been shown to be cytoprotective against thermal injury in rats. This approach has not yet been tested in domestic animals. Likewise, treatment of lactating dairy cows with bovine somatotropin has been shown to increase evaporative heat loss capacity. Understanding the molecular basis for the increased evaporative heat loss capability offers new opportunities for increasing thermal tolerance of cattle in warm climates. Cataloging molecular changes associated with seasonal adaptation will also offer new insights into selecting domestic animals for thermal tolerance.

Table 4. Candidate genes for thermal resistance.

Gene	Species	Reference
Hsp 70.1[1]	mouse	Huang et al., 2001
Hsp 70.3[2]	mouse	Huang et al., 2001
Hsp 72	human	Fehrenbach et al., 2001
Oxt[3]	mouse	Wesolowski et al., 2003.
Timp-2[4]	mouse	Wesolowski et al., 2003
Rpl3[5]	mouse	Wesolowski et al., 2003
Slick Gene	cattle	Olsen et al., 2003
Kit locus[6]	cattle	Reinsch et al., 1999

1. Heat shock protein 70.1
2. Heat shock protein 70.3
3. Oxytocin
4. Tissue inhibitor of metalloproteinase 2
5. Ribosmal protein L3
6. Receptor tyrosine kinase

Conclusions

Advent of new tools in molecular biology as well as the opportunity to follow dynamic changes in the core and surface temperature of domestic animals permits the first thorough evaluation of the effect of environmental temperature on gene expression. To date, only a few genes have been identified as potential candidates for manipulation to improve thermotolerance. Care will need to be taken to avoid confounding changes in gene expression associated with acclimation with those associated with adaptation. A thorough understanding of the coordination of gene function in response to thermal stress will also need to be understood before specific genetic manipulations can be expected to be productive. For example, many of the coordinated responses to acute thermal stress are deleterious to production. However, there are indications that improving heat loss mechanisms may allow animals to remain productive during periods of high environmental heat load.

References

Bauman, D.E., 2000. Regulation of nutrient partitioning during lactation: homeostasis and homeorhesis revisited. In: Rumen Physiology: Digestion, Metabolism, Growth and Reproduction. Edited by P.J. Cronje. CAB Publishing, New York, NY. 311-327.

Becker, B.A., H.D. Johnson, R.L. & R.J. Collier, 1990. Effect of farm and simulated laboratory cold environmental conditions on the performance and physiological responses of lactating dairy cows supplemented with bovine somatotropin. Int. J. Biomet.34: 151-156.

Beede, D.K. & R.J. Collier, 1986.Potential nutritional strategies for intensively managed cattle during thermal stress. J. Anim. Sci. 62: 543-554.

Bligh, J., 1976. Introduction to acclamatory adaptation-including notes on terminology. In: Environmental Physiology of Animals. Ed. J. Bligh, J.L. Cloudsley-Thompson and A. G. McDonald. John Wiley & Sons, New York, NY. Pp.219-229.

Christian. G.I. & H.D. Johnson, 1972. Cortisol turnover in heat-stressed cows. J. Anim. Sci. 32: 1005-1010.

Collier, R.J., D.K. Beede, W.W. Thatcher, L.A. Israel & C.J. Wilcox, 1982. Influences of environment and its modification on dairy animal health and production. J. Dairy Sci. 65: 2213-2227.

Collier, R.J., S.G. Doelger, H.H. Head, W. W. Thatcher & C.J. Wilcox, 1982. Effects of heat stress during pregnancy on maternal hormone concentrations, calf birth weight and postpartum milk yield of Holstein cows. J. Anim. Sci. 54: 309-319.

Esmay, M.L., 1978. Principles of Animal Environment. Textbook Edition. AVI Publishing Company, Inc. Westport, Conn.

Fehrenbach, E., A.M. Niess, R. Veith, H.H. Dickhuth & H. Northoff, 2001. Changes of HSP-72 expression in leukocytes are associated with adaptation to exercise under conditions of high environmental temperature. J. Leuckocyte Biol. 69:747-754.

Horowitz, M., M.J. Peiser & A. Muhlrad, 1986. Alterations in cardiac myosin distribution as an adaptation to chronic environmental stress. J. Mol. Cell. Cardiol. 18:511-515.

Horowitz, M., 2001 Heat acclimation: phenotypic plasticity and cues to the underlying molecular mechanisms. J Thermal Biol. 26:357-363.

Huang, L., N.F. Mivechi & D. Moskophidis, 2001. Insights into regulation and function of the major stress-induced hsp70 molecular chaperone in Vivo: Analysis of mice with targeted gene disruption of the hsp70.1 or hsp70.3 gene. Molec and Cell. Biol. 21:8575-8591.

Keister, Z.O., K.D. Moss, H.M. Zhang, T. Teegerstrom, R.A. Edling, R.J. Collier & R.L. Ax, 2002. Physiological responses in thermal stressed Jersey cows subjected to different management strategies. J Dairy Sci. 85:3217-3224.

Lefcourt, A.M., & W.R. Adams, 1996. Radiotelemetry measurement of body temperatures of feedlot steers during summer. J. Anim. Sci. 74:2633-2640.

Lemerle, C. & M.E. Goddard, 1986. Assessment of heat stress in dairy cattle in Papua, New Guinea. Trop. Anim. Hlth. Prod. 18:232-242.

McVicker, L.E., M.J. Leonard & D.E. Spiers, 2002. Evaluation of feedlot cattle response to summer heat in open or shaded pens. Proc. 15th Conf. Biomet and Aerobiol. 104-105.

Manulu, W., H.D. Johnson, R.Z. Li, B.A. Becker & R.J. Collier, 1991. Assessment of thermal status of somatotropin-injected lactating Holstein cows maintained under controlled-laboratory thermoneutral, hot and cold environments. J. Nutri.121.:2006-2019.

Moraes, V.M.B., R.D. Malheiro, V. Bruggeman, A. Collin, K. Tona, P. Van As, O.M. Onagbesan, J. Buyse, E. Decuypere & M. Macari, 2003. Effect of thermal conditioning during embryonic development on aspects of physiological responses of broilers to heat stress. J. Thermal Biol. 28:133-140.

Nienaber J.A. & G.L. Hahn, 1991. Associations among body temperature, eating and heat production in swine and cattle. Proc.12th Symp. On Energy Metabolism in Farm Animals. Switzerland, Sept 1-7, EAAP Pub No 58:458-461.

Nienaber, J.A., G.L. Hahn & R.A. Eigenberg, 1999. Quantifying livestock responses for heat stress management: a review. Int. J. Biometerol. 42:183-188.

Olsen, T.A., C. Lucena, C.C. Chase Jr. & A.C. Hammond, 2003. Evidence of a major gne influencing hair length and heat tolerance in Bos Taurus cattle. J. Anim. Sci. 81:80-90.

Ravagnolo, O., I. Mistzal & G. Hoogenboom, 2000. Genetic component of heat stress in cattle, development of a heat index function. J. Dairy Sci. 83:2120-2125.

Ravagnolo, O. & I. Misztal, 2002. Studies on genetics of heat tolerance in dairy cattle with reduced weather information via cluster analysis. J. Dairy Sci. 85:1586-1589.

Ray, D.E., T.J. Halbach & D.V. Armstrong, 1992. Season and lactation number effects on milk production and reproduction of dairy cattle in Arizona. J. Dairy Sci. 75:2976-2983.

Reinsch, N., H. X. N. Thomsen, M. Brink, C. Loof, E. Kalm, G.A. Brockman, S. Grupe, C.Kuhn, M. Schwerin, B. Leyhe, S. Hiendleder, G., Erhardt, I. Medjugorac, I. Russ, M. Forster, R. Reents & G. Averdunk, 1999. A QTL for the degree of spotting in cattle shows synteny with the KIT locus on chromosome 6. J. Hered. 6:629-634.

SAS User's Guide: Statistics. 1996. SAS Institute Inc., Cary, NC.

Statview, 1998. Statview Reference. SAS Institute Inc. Cary, NC.

Thatcher, W.W., 1974. Effects of season, climate and temperature on reproduction and lactation. J. Dairy Sci. 57:360-368.

Wesolowski, S.R., M.F. Allan, M.K. Nielsen & D. Pomp, 2003. Evaluation of hypothalamic gene expression in mice. Physiol. Genomics. 10:1152-1187.

Wolfgram, A.L., Y. Kobayashi & R.J. Collier, 2003. Assessment of infrared thermometry and thermography to evaluate heat stress in lactating dairy cattle.

J. Dairy Sci. (submitted).

Zwald, N.R., K.A. Weigel, W.F. Fikse & R. Rekaya, 2003. Identification of factors that cause genotype by environment interaction between herds of Holstein cattle in seventeen countries. J. Dairy Sci. 86:1009-1018.

Contribution of animal husbandry to climatic changes

J. Hartung

Institute for Animal Hygiene, Animal Welfare and Behaviour of Farm Animals, School of Veterinary Medicine Hanover, Bünteweg 17 P, 30559 Hanover, Germany, itt@tiho-hannover.de

Summary

Animal husbandry systems are the source of a large variety of different gases which can be both a nuisance and environmentally harmful. The most important greenhouse gases are methane (CH_4) and nitrous oxide (N_2O). Relative to carbon dioxide (CO_2), the amounts of CH_4 and N_2O in the atmosphere are low, but their global warming potential (GWP) is 21 and 310 times higher than that of CO_2, respectively. The total global emissions are estimated at 535 Tg (CH_4) and 17.7 Tg (N_2O) per year. About 45 % of the methane production originates from agriculture, and nearly 20 % comes from animal production. N_2O emission from anthropogenic sources is around 8 Tg per year and, of these, 6.2 Tg come from livestock production. There are substantial uncertainties in all of these estimates because there are large variations in emission rates mainly due to the many influencing factors such as temperature or substrate or keeping conditions. While emission amounts of CH_4 from ruminants are relatively well known there is a considerable lack of knowledge for other species. Similarly, the reliability of the N_2O data is still poor. Animal production systems which use straw seem to release distinct higher amounts of N_2O than those employing liquid manure systems. This may result in conflicts with welfare policies introducing animal friendly and littered keeping systems. It seems necessary to enhance more detailed research in sources and sinks of these gases and that the national and international emission inventories are regularly up-dated in the light of new findings.

Keywords: global warming, methane, nitrous oxide, animal husbandry

Introduction

Modern livestock production is increasingly regarded as a source of solid, liquid and airborne emissions which can be both a nuisance and environmentally harmful. Solid and liquid manure and waste water contain nitrogen and phosphorus which are the most important plant nutrients, but are harmful when applied to agricultural land in excess amounts thereby leading to pollution of ground water by nitrates and surface water by phosphorous causing eutrophication. The soil can also be polluted with heavy metals such as zinc and copper which are used as growth promoters in the feed stuff of farm animals, and by a group of potentially hazardous effluents such as drug residues (e.g. antibiotics), which may be present in the excreta of farm animals after medical treatment and which are passed to the environment during grazing or spreading of animal manure where they may conceivably contribute to the formation of antibiotic resistance in certain strains of bacteria (Hartung & Wathes, 2001).
The most important aerial pollutants are odours, gases, dust, micro-organisms and compounds such as endotoxins, together also called bioaerosols, which are emitted by way of the exhaust air into the environment from buildings and during manure storage, handling and disposal as well as grazing. Between 136 (Hartung, 1992) and 203 (Schiffman et al., 2001) different gaseous compounds have been identified in the atmosphere of various animal houses, which are a major source of these pollutants. Aerial pollutants can give cause for concern for several

reasons. Firstly, there is strong epidemiological evidence that the health of farmers working in animal houses may be harmed by regular occupational exposure to air pollutants. Various reviews demonstrate the consequences of poor air hygiene for the respiratory health of farmers (Whythe, 1993; Donham, 1993; Radon et al., 2002). Secondly, an animal's respiratory health may be compromised by these pollutants. In some herds, half of all slaughter pigs may show signs of pneumonia, pleuritis or other respiratory disease (von Altrock, 1998). Thirdly, many of the above mentioned gases are odorous and can cause odour pollution in the vicinity of farm animal enterprises bringing about legal complaints of nearby residents. Fourthly, there are suggestions that particulate emissions, such as dust and micro-organisms, from livestock buildings may be harmful for people living close to livestock buildings. A recent survey is given by Seedorf & Hartung (2002). The fifth reason for concern is that ammonia (NH_3) emitted from animal manure can damage trees directly, forms precursors of secondary aerosols in the atmosphere and contributes to soil acidification (Jarvis & Pain, 1990; Jarvis, 2002). Table 1 gives a brief overview on the most important pollutants emitted from livestock production and its impact on farm livestock, man and the environment.

Table 1. Environmental impact from livestock sources.

Substance/Compound	Impact on people	Impact on animals	Impact on ecology	Local	Regional	Global
Odour	nuisance	no	no	yes	(yes)	no
Ammonia NH_3	indoors irritant	high irritant	high nutrient	high direct	yes PM 2.5+SOx	low
Hydrogen sulphide H_2S	indoors toxic	indoors toxic	no	odour	no	no
Methane CH_4	no explosive	no global warming	yes global warming	NO	(no)	yes
Nitrous oxide N_2O	no	no	high global warming	low	low	yes
Dust	allergy?	health	low	yes	(PM 10)	no
Bacteria/Virus	infection	infections	low	yes	yes?	no?
Endotoxins	yes	yes	no	yes	(yes)	no
Nitrate/Nitrite	drinking water	no	eutrophication	yes	(yes)	no
Phosphate			eutrophication	yes	yes	no
Copper/Zinc	low pig liver	yes sheep!	yes soil	yes	yes	no
Vet drugs	resistance?	resistance?	?	?	?	?

Far less attention was paid for a long time to the fact, that livestock and its manure are also a major source of atmospheric pollutants such as methane (CH_4) nitrous oxide (N_2O) and carbon dioxide (CO_2), which are strong "green house gases" enhancing global warming (van Amstel, 1993). The reason for the relatively low recognition was probably due to the low health risks for animal and man associated with these gases. Methane and nitrous oxide contribute to the greenhouse effect, but do not cause problems indoors or outdoors for farm workers or animals.

The increase of the atmospheric concentrations of greenhouse gases, typically methane, nitrous oxide and carbon dioxide, is significant over the last decades and about 20% of global methane production is suggested to originate from ruminants (Williams, 1994). Apart from increasing gas intakes into the atmosphere the accumulation of greenhouse gases is dramatically caused by their long individual lifetime (Table 2), which is defined as the burden divided by the mean global sink for a gas in steady state (i.e., with unchanging production). Changes in atmospheric composition and chemistry over the past century have additionally affected the lifetimes of many greenhouse gases (IPCC 2001).

Table 2. Characteristics for selected greenhouse gases including atmospheric concentrations, yearly rate of change and lifetimes.

Substance/Compound	CO_2	CH_4	N_2O
Pre-industrial concentration	280 ppm	700 ppb	270 ppb
Concentration in 1998	365 ppm	1745 ppb	314 ppb
Rate of change	1.5 ppm per year	7.0 ppb per year	0.8 ppb per year
Atmospheric lifetime	5-200 years	12 years	114 years

Source: McBean et al. (2001)

The aim of this paper is to briefly summarise the emission potential of the two most relevant greenhouse gases associated with livestock production, methane and nitrous oxide. Because of the complex nature of animal farming emission factors are given for the different species and housing systems. Aspects of mitigation and the relation to other areas of animal protection are discussed.

Mechanisms of production

Methane

Enteric fermentation is the main reason for methane generation in the digestive systems of animals. Generally, the higher the feed intake, the higher the methane emission. Feed intake is positively related to animal size, growth rate and production (e.g. milk produktion, wool growth, pregnancy). The type of digestive system has a significant influence on the rate of methane release. Ruminant animals with a polygastric digestion system (cattle, buffalo, goats, sheep, camels, deers) have the highest emission potential because microbial-related anaerobic degradation processes of the fodder are responsible for the methane production in the rumen. The intra-gastrical produced methane is then finally discharged into the ambient air caused by the eructation through the oesophagus.

In contrast to the polygastric animals, monogastric animals (swine) have relatively low methane emissions because much less methane producing fermentation takes place in their digestive system. The pathway into the atmosphere is mainly caused by flatulence.

The second considerable source is the manure. Livestock manure management has a considerable impact on methane emissions. Livestock manure is principally composed of organic material. When this organic material decomposes in an anaerobic environment, methanogenic bacteria produce methane. This process is mainly due to liquid manure storage in tanks, pits or lagoons. Important factors influencing methanogenesis are the amount and surface area of the manure, ambient and core manure temperature and the strength and frequency of manure agitation, which forces more aerobic processes with lower methane emissions, for instance (Hartung & Monteny, 2000).

Nitrous oxide

Nitrous oxide is produced by bacterial processes in manure which allows composting processes. It is somewhat a secondary reaction product of primary nitrogen compounds which are decomposed by the dynamic processes of nitrification and denitrification. Such a primary compound is dissolved ammonia (NH_4^+), which interacts with nitrifying bacteria (*Nitrosomonas* spp., *Nitrobacter* spp.) under aerobic conditions according to the equation:

$$NH_4^+ \rightarrow NO_2^- \rightarrow NO_3^- \quad (1)$$

Under optimal oxygen conditions, nitrification does not cause the formation of nitrous oxide as an intermediate product. Ammonium or ammonia are transformed to nitrate. Under ideal conditions this may happen in deep-litter systems. Microbial processes enhance composting. Aerobic bacterial degradation causes heat production which is of hygienic importance. Deep-litter systems are, however, complex systems with a large variation in space, time type and amount of litter. Gradients exist in the litter bed, e.g. oxygen decreases with depth and also in aggregates. Aerobic processes can predominantly occur near the surface of the bed and of the aggregates. Low oxygen and anoxic processes will take place in the deeper layers. Sub-optimal conditions with low available oxygen can enhance the reduction of oxidized nitrogen compounds. As a result, the nitrification process is incomplete and considerable amounts of nitrous oxide are accumulated and released as an artefact or side effect. That seems to happen in deep litter systems and to a much smaller extent in liquid manure systems
Denitrification is a kind of chain reaction with several reaction steps and different in-between products. Starting with nitrate the process involves the generation of nitrite, nitrogen oxide, nitrous oxide and finally pure nitrogen. By denitrification large amounts of nitrate can be turned in harmless genuine nitrogen. Equation 2 shows the principle of the transformation.

$$NO_{3-} \rightarrow NO_{2-} \rightarrow NO \rightarrow N_2O \rightarrow N_2 \quad (2)$$

Nitrates formed under aerobic conditions will be transformed by microbial denitrification when the oxygen pressure is low. However, a low carbon-to-nitrogen ratio (C:N) as e.g. in pig wastes makes it difficult to transform surplus ammonia into microbial cells. The formation of nitrous oxide depends on the access of oxygen. This oxygen supply varies in the different manure management and handling systems and is determined by bedding, storage conditions and other factors. Typically liquid manure is not causing significant amounts of nitrous oxide, because of the anaerobic conditions as long as the manure is not stirred up. In deep litter systems semi-aerobic conditions are present with poor oxygen availabilities and the above described nitrous oxide formation processes occur in considerable amounts (Hartung & Monteny, 2000; Groenestein et al., 1993).

Carbon dioxide

Carbon dioxide is part of the global carbon cycle and have been severely disbalanced by anthropogenic actions. The largest change comes from the combustion of fossil fuels, what produce carbon dioxide in a magnitude, which cannot be sufficiently immobilized by growing biomass. Additionally, the increasing worldwide deforestation reduce potential sinks for carbon dioxide. Therefore, the contribution of animal farming to the currently observed increase of carbon dioxide concentration in the atmosphere is very low

Emissions from livestock production

The described mechanisms of greenhouse gas generation in animal production contribute in quite different extents to the climatic change process. The main greenhouse gas CO_2 plays no role in the agricultural sector. With a proportion of 0.03 % of the total European wide CO_2 emission this gas can be neglected (EEA 2001a,b). But methane from agriculture is the main contributor to the gaseous atmospheric pollution. Emissions of 8.527 kilotonnes (kt) in 1998 caused nearly 50 % of the overall released methane quantities in Europe and is addressed mainly to ruminant animals (EEA 2001c). The percentage of agriculture-related nitrous oxide is even still higher than for CH_4. An emitted quantity of 701 kt in 1998 constitutes a portion of 61 % in relation to all relevant sectors. But in contrast to methane and its generation in animals, organic and synthetic fertiliser use and leguminous crops are the dominant targets in N_2O production (EEA, 2001d). As consequence, agricultural soils are generally the most effective N_2O emission surfaces. This can be clearly seen if soil- and livestock manure-related emission quantities are compared. In a global scale, which considered the so called developed countries, the former emission source caused 2,080 kt, but manure was responsible for 277 kt only. In the same year 2000, the methane emission caused by livestock enteric fermentation and manure management caused 25,100 and 4,930 kt worldwide, respectively (EPA 2001).

Due to their strong effect in climate changes, researchers and policy makers are seeking for valid emission factors, which enables them to design inventories, future scenarios of climate changes and targets of greenhouse gas reduction goals. Therefore, in the livestock sector there is a great demand on species-related emission factors, expressed as mass per animal place and year. Although limiting factors in the methodology are causing uncertainties (i.e. different usable measurement techniques and strategies, diurnal and seasonal variation of emission rates) a relative widespread database exists for the most common livestock species like cattle, pigs and poultry (Hartung & Monteny, 2000; Hartung, 2001). This data base is a very useful tool to build on. However, there are still considerable gaps when sheep are not considered as methane emitters in Europe, although in other parts of the world these small ruminants contribute to 58 % of the total methane emission compared to 28% from beef cattle and 18 % from dairy cattle (MAF 1993). Some selected basic emission factors are shown in Table 3.

Table 3. Greenhouse gas emissions from animal production facilities.

Species	CH_4 - enteric fermentation[1] kg animal^{-1} y^{-1}	CH_4 -manure kg animal^{-1} y^{-1}	N_2O kg animal^{-1} y^{-1}
Cattle (Dairy)	100	345	0.8 g LU^{-1} d^{-1} [(2)]
Pigs	1	32	0.15[3]
Poultry	0.1	2.4	0.017[4]

[1]UBA, 2001; [2]Sneath et al., 1997; [3]Fattening pigs on fully slatted floors (Hahne et al., 1999); [4]Laying hens, floor system with straw (Mennicken, 1998)

Conclusions

- Livestock farming causes significant emissions of greenhouse gases such as methane and nitrous oxide.
- The formation and emission of these gases is based on very complex biological processes and technical conditions.

- Most of the methane emissions originate from ruminants. The second largest source are manure stores.
- Methane is mainly a primary product of anaerobic processes.
- Nitrous oxide is formed as a secondary reaction product under non-optimal conditions in litter when nitrification and denitrification do not run to completion.
- There are available only limited precise emission rates for methane and nitrous oxide from the large variety of animal species and husbandry systems.
- More detailed research is needed to verify and deepen the present knowledge. This concerns agricultural engineers, animal scientists, nutritionists, veterinarians and environmentalists.

Recommendations

1. The instrumentation for the measurement of these gases should be improved to meet minimum requirements acceptable in all countries in order to be able to compare results from different working groups.
2. An accepted measuring protocol is needed to standardise analytical procedures in terms of measurement cycles, time of the day, duration of single measurements, number and form of repetitions.
3. This is particularly necessary for the measurement of nitrous oxide which occurs often in very low concentrations only.
4. The calculation factors presently used should be regularly updated in the light of new knowledge.
5. At the same time nutritionists are asked to develop adequate and efficient feeding regimes with minimal wastage of nitrogen and low methane production.
6. The development of low emission production systems should be encouraged including mitigation techniques, eg. biofilters, bioscrubbers, covered manure pits and shallow manure application.
7. It is also necessary to take as early as possible into account the need of the farm animals for animal friendly keeping systems when new low emitting husbandry systems are going to be developed.
8. Future oriented, sustainable housing and keeping systems for farm animals have to consider beside the protection of the environment the needs of the animals (health and welfare) and the consumer who can expect safe and wholesome food of animal origin.
9. An environmental risk analysis is required to compare different production systems and different regions in the world particularly in respect to greenhouse gases.
10. Standards for animal production should be established and applied to all European countries observing the sometimes apparently conflicting areas for the sake of consumers, the environment and the animals.
11. For the realization of these aims the cooperation of farmers, agricultural engineers, veterinarians and governmental agencies is necessary.

Acknowledgement

The author thanks Dr. Eberhard Hartung, University of Hohenheim, Germany and Dr. Jens Seedorf, School of Veterinary Medicine Hanover, Germany for providing important literature information.

References

Altrock, von, A., 1998. Untersuchungen zum Vorkommen bakterieller Infektionserreger in pathologisch-anatomisch veränderten Lungen von Schweinen und Zusammenstellung der Resistenzspektren. Berl. Münch. Tierärztl. Wschr., 111, 164-172.

Amstel, A. R., van, 1993. Methane and nitrous oxide: methods in national emission inventories and options for control. Proc. Internat. IPCC Workshop, Amerfoort, Netherlands

Donham, K.J., 1993. Respiratory disease hazards to workers in livestock and poultry confined structures. Sem. Respir. Med., 14, 49-59.

EEA, 2001a. Total EU greenhouse gas emission. European Environment Agency, Factsheets, http://themes.eea.eu.int/Environmental_issues/climate/indicators/Kyoto_Protocol_targets/yir99cc5.pdf

EEA, 2001b. Total EU CO_2 emissions. European Environment Agency, Factsheets, http://themes.eea.eu.int/Environmental_issues/climate/indicators/Carbon_dioxide_emissions/yir99cc1.pdf

EEA, 2001c. Total EU CH_4 emissions. European Environment Agency, Factsheets, http://themes.eea.eu.int/Environmental_issues/climate/indicators/methane_emission/yir99cc2.pdf

EEA, 2001d. Total EU N_2O emissions. European Environment Agency, Factsheets, http://themes.eea.eu.int/Environmental_issues/climate/indicators/nitrous_oxide_emissions/yir99cc3.pdf

EPA, 2001. Non-CO2 Greenhouse Gas Emissions from Developed Countries: 1990-2010. Environmental Protection Agency, Office of Air and Radiation, Washington, USA. http://www.epa.gov/ghginfo/pdfs/r1_new/fulldocument.pdf

Groenestein, C.M., J. Oosthoek & H.G. van Faassen 1993. Microbial processes in deep litter systems for fattening pigsand emission of ammonia, nitrous oxide and nitric oxide. In: „Nitrogen flow in pig productionan environmental consequences“. Proc. 1st International Symposium. Wageningen, NL. June 8-11, p. 269-274.

Hahne, J., D. Hesse & K.D. Vorlop 1999. Spurengasemissionen aus der Mastschweinehaltung. Landtechnik, 54, 180-181.

Hartung, E. 2001. Greenhouse gas emissions from animal husbandry. In: J. Hartung & C.M. Wathes (eds.) Livestock Farming and the Environment. Landbauforschung Special Issue 226, p. 5-10.

Hartung, E. & G.J. Monteny 2000. Methane (CH4) and nitrous oxide (N2O) emissions from animal husbandry. Agrartechn. Forsch., 6, E62-E69.

Hartung, J. 1992. Gas- und partikelförmige Emissionen aus Nutztierställen. Pneumologie 46, 196-202

IPCC, 2001. Climate Change 2001: A Scientific Basis, Intergovernmental Panel on Climate Change; J.T. Houghton, Y. Ding, D.J. Griggs, M. Noguer, P.J. van der Linden, X. Dai, C.A. Johnson, and K. Maskell, eds.; Cambridge University Press. Cambridge, U.K.

Jarvis, S. C. 2002. Environmental impacts of cattle housing and grazing. In: Kaske et al. (eds.) Recent developments and perspectives in bovine medicine. Keynote lectures, Proc. 12th World Buiatric Congress, 18-23 August, 2003, Hannover, p. 11-23

Jarvis, S. C. & B. F. Pain 1990. Ammonia volatilisation from agricultural land. Proc. Fertilizer Society, Peterborough, UK, 298

MAF, 1993. Greenhouse gas emission policies: Impact on agriculture. Policy Technical Paper 93/6, Ministry of Agriculture and Forestry, New Zealand. http://www.maf.govt.nz/mafnet/rural-nz/sustainable-resource-use/climate/greenhouse-gas-policies/greengas-14.htm#P1528_139751

McBean, G., A. Weaver & N. Roulet 2001. The science of climate change: What do we know ? Can. J. Policy Res., 2, 16-25.

Mennicken, L., 1998. Biobett für Legehennen - ein Beitrag zum Umweltschutz ? DGS, 13, 12-20.

Radon, K., E. Monso, C. Weber, B. Dauser, M. Iversen, U. Opravil, K. Donham, J. Hartung, S. Pedersen, S. Garz, D. Blainey, U. Rabe & D. Nowak 2002. Prevalence and risk factors for airway diseases in farmers – summary of results of the european farmers′ project. Ann Agric Environ Med 9, 207-213

Schiffman, S. S., J. L. Benett & J. H. Raymer 2001. Quantification of odors and odorants from swine operations in North Carolina. Agri. Forest Meteorol., 108, 213-240.

Seedorf, J. & J. Hartung 2002. Stäube und Mikroorganismen in der Tierhaltung. KTBL-Schrift 393, Landwirtschaftsverlag GmbH, Münster, 166 Seiten.

Sneath, R. W., V. R. Phillips, T. G. M. Demmers, L. R. Burgess, J. L. Short & S. K. Welch 1997. Long term measurments of greenhouse gas emissions from UK livestock buildings. Livestock Environment V, Proc. 5th Int. Symp., Bloomington, Minnesota, USA, 146-153.

UBA, 2001. Erstellung eines Gutachtens für einen deutschen Beitrag zur Vollzugsvorbereitung zur Umsetzung der IVU-Richtlinie für den Bereich Intensivtierhaltung. Umweltbundesamt, Vorhaben FKZ 36008001, Berlin, Germany

Whythe, R. T. 1993. Aerial pollutants and the health of poultry farmers. World's Poultry Science Journal, 49, 139-156

Williams, A.G., 1994. Methane emissions. Report No. 28, London, Watt Committee.

Strategies for reducing the effects of animal husbandry on climate

G.J. Monteny

Institute of Agricultural and Environmental Engineering (IMAG), POBox 43, NL-6700 AA Wageningen, The Netherlands, gert-jan.monteny@wur.nl

Summary

Animal production considerably contributes to the emissions of methane and nitrous oxide. Both gases contribute to global warming. Insight into the processes and influencing factors that play a role in the production and transport of these gases is essential to identify strategies for abatement of their emissions. Methane is mainly produced from enteric fermentation and its production is strongly related with the animal diet. It is also produced from animal manures, depending on manure composition, temperature, presence of bacteria and pH. Nitrous oxide originates from nitrogen related processes nitrification and de-nitrification, and its production greatly depends on the nitrogen pressure, soil conditions and the availability of an energy source (carbon). Because of their poor solubility in water, the methane and nitrous oxide produced will easily be transported to the atmosphere, so reducing measures at the source or 'beginning of pipe' have to be considered. Most important ways to reduce methane emissions is through dietary measures (e.g. reducing the amount of roughage), by adapting the housing system (innovative floor systems, resulting in separation of faeces and urine), manure management (cooling), manure treatment (e.g. acidification), and air purification (bio-filters). Nitrous oxide emissions can be reduced by pasture and fertilization management, resulting in a reduction of the nitrogen pressure, and herd management (restricted grazing). Because of the difference in the origin of methane (carbon cycle) and nitrous oxide (nitrogen cycle), interactions between their emissions and between options for mitigation of other pollutant emissions (ammonia, nitrate) have to be taken into account.

Keywords: methane, nitrous oxide, biogas, composting, economy, global warming, cattle, pigs, poultry, manure, fertilizers, environmental pollution

Introduction

The number of animals kept on farms for the production of milk and dairy products, meat and eggs has increased during the past century, in order to feed the growing world population. In global regions like Western Europe and Northern America, this increase was speeded by the introduction of concentrates and chemical fertilizers after the second world war, which also led to specialization and intensification of animal production. Nowadays, FAO-data clearly show a stabilization of or even a decrease in the numbers of livestock in these regions, whereas growing animal numbers are reported in developing regions like China.

Increasing animal numbers and use of natural resources have resulted in a diversity of environmental pollution issues. Odour nuisance may be the oldest pollution aspect associated with intensive animal production. Ground and surface water pollution, upon excessive use and losses of nitrogen and phosphate from animal and chemical manures, and environmental acidification and eutrophication related to the emission and deposition of ammonia (NH_3) have gained importance during the past decades. Of more recent date is the awareness of the contribution of animal husbandry to the problem of global warming. In this perspective,

emissions of the non-CO_2 greenhouse gases methane (CH_4) and nitrous oxide (N_2O) are playing a key role.
This paper briefly addresses developments in animal numbers in a global perspective, and the environmental issues associated, with emphasis on the greenhouse gases CH_4 and N_2O. The processes and factors that play a role in the production and the emission of both gases are used to present and discuss options and strategies for reduction of the impact on global warming. In this perspective, conclusions are drawn on the most effective way to reduce greenhouse gas emissions and some important non-technical dimensions associated. This paper is mainly based upon European research into the emission and abatement of non-CO_2 greenhouse gases. No attention is paid to the indirect emissions of greenhouse gases e.g. due to transportation.

Animal husbandry and global warming in brief

Recent estimates of the annual global emissions of CH_4 and N_2O are 535 and 18 Mton, respectively (Houghton et al., 1996; Kroeze et al.; 1999). In table 1, the relative contributions of natural sources and anthropogenic sources, including animal husbandry are presented.

Table 1. Relative contribution of various sources to the global emission of non-CO_2 greenhouse gases.

	Natural sources	Anthropogenic sources	
		Animal husbandry	Others
CH_4	30	20	50
N_2O	55	35	10

These data show that anthropogenic sources are the most important for the global emission of CH_4, whereas natural and anthropogenic sources are almost equally important for N_2O. Important anthropogenic sources of CH_4 emissions are the burning of biomass and rice production. Animal husbandry related sources are mainly the digestion system of ruminants and animal excreta. Moreover, animal husbandry largely accounts for the anthropogenic emission of N_2O, which is strongly related to the use of chemical and animal fertilizers. Emissions of CH_4 and N_2O on a European level amounted 19.4 and 1.9 Mton per year in 1990 (Brink et al., 2001), respectively, and tend to decrease significantly due to reduced amounts of chemical fertilisers used and livestock numbers.
The contribution of N_2O to global warming is well described and severe (320 times the CO_2 Global Warming Potential = GWP), but also CH4 (GWP = 21) is a major contributor. Also, N_2O emissions contribute to depletion of ozone in the stratosphere, via stratospheric conversion of N_2O to nitrogen oxides (NO) (Olivier et al., 1998).

Methane and nitrous oxide: processes and influencing factors

Insight into the processes and influencing factors that play a role in the production and transport CH_4 and N_2O helps to identify strategies for emission abatement. These strategies may be technical or technological, management related or both. They can interfere at the 'beginning of pipe, or at the source, at intermediate stages (enclosures, like the manure pit or the outdoor storage), or at the 'end of pipe', at the boundaries of the emitting surface areas and the atmosphere.

Gas sources ('beginning of pipe')

Methane and nitrous oxide are produced as gaseous reaction products of different nutrient cycles, namely the carbon (C) and the nitrogen (N) cycle, respectively. Moreover, CH_4 results from anoxic or anaerobic decomposition processes, whereas N_2O is mainly produced in an environment were oxygen is present (aerobic processes). It is, therefore, obvious that the processes and influencing factors for their production and release (= emission) differ strongly. Methane is mainly produced as a by-product of the fermentation of the digestible organic matter in the diet, and especially during the carbon hydrate fermentation. The ruminant digestion system (rumen) is a complex system of various micro organisms (see e.g. Nolan, 1999). In the rumen, hydrogen (H_2) needs to be eliminated to avoid negative feed back effects on fermentation. The production of CH_4 is the most effective pathway to achieve this. Forage based diets stimulate acetate and CH_4 production, whereas cereal based diets enhance propionate production at the expense of CH_4. The diet composition, therefore, is an important influencing factor.
Manure is also a significant source of CH_4. The remainder of digestible organic matter in the feces may be hydrolyzed (anaerobic digestion) during storage, either inside or outside the animal house. This process is well described by Zeeman (1991). Most important factors that determine the rate of CH_4 production from manure are: manure composition (organic matter content or amount of volatile solids), temperature, presence of methanogenic bacteria and pH.

Nitrous oxide is produced as a result of nitrification and de-nitrification (see process equations 1 and 2).

Nitrification: $$NH_4^+ \xrightarrow{\text{Nitrosomonas spp.}} NO_2^- \xrightarrow{\text{Nitrobacter spp}} NO_3^- \quad (1)$$

De-nitrification: $$NO_3^- \rightarrow NO_2^- \rightarrow NO \rightarrow N_2O \rightarrow N_2 \quad (2)$$

These processes occur in the soil and in beddings in animal houses, as well as during composting of manure and in organic coverings of manure storages. The quality of these processes in soils, and thus the quantity of N_2O produced, greatly depends on the N fertilization level, the ground water table and the soil properties. Soils that are rich with organic matter have a greater N_2O production potential than soils that with low organic matter content. Furthermore, N_2O production increases with the soil moisture content (reduced oxygen). In straw or litter based housing and storage (e.g. composting) systems, similar to the soil, the partially aerobic conditions enhance nitrification, whereas the availability of a energy source (carbon) is important for de-nitrification. The amount of N_2O produced greatly depends on N loading, dry matter content (microbial activity) and oxygen situation (related to the measure of compaction of the bedding material).

Intermediate processes

Different than for ammonia (NH_3), being another important polluting emission from agriculture, CH_4 and N_2O are poorly soluble in water, and thus in watery solutions like manure. Monteny (2000) describes the NH_3 related processes and concludes that a relatively small percentage of the NH_3 produced from urea conversion will emit to the atmosphere during housing and storage. The vast majority is released after land spreading of manure in the field. The high water solubility is the critical process, with pH and temperature as the most important influencing factors. This means that lowering of pH and temperature, with a reduced amount of free NH_3 in the solution, are effective measures to reduce NH_3 emissions.

No such relationships are at stake for the greenhouse gases considered. This means that all CH_4 and N_2O produced will directly be transported in the manure, soil or bedding (diffusion), and volatilize (convective mass transfer) to the air above the manure. The same holds for CH_4 produced in the animal digestion system, where the CH_4 produced is released from the animal through breath and flatus. Consequently, abatement through intermediate processes can only be realized if mixing of ambient air with gas polluted air can be avoided.

End of pipe

End of pipe solutions should focus on preventing polluted air or the gases considered from being released into the atmosphere. This is hard to accomplish in animal buildings, since ventilation is operated to remove CO_2, water vapor and temperature control, and for soils, where a free exchange of air between pores and atmosphere exists. For outdoor stored manure, separating polluted air from the ambient air can prevent polluted air release. This will, however, only be of temporary value since manure is used on farms for fertilization purposes and has to be removed from the stores. Gas removal, therefore, seems to be the most important process to prevent greenhouse gas emissions.

Strategies for reduction of methane and nitrous oxide

Possible strategies for reducing emissions of CH_4 and N_2O will have to based upon the processes and influencing factors presented in the previous section. Besides, the relative importance of each of the sources and their accessibility with have to be taken into account.

Dietary measures

Veen (2001) made an inventory of the cattle diet related measures to reduce CH_4 emissions. He concluded that replacement of roughage by concentrates and improvement of feed conversion efficiency (e.g. by including more non-structural carbon hydrates in the diet) were the most feasible in practice. Base on his findings, CH_4 production from grass and maize based diets amounted 24 g per kg of dry matter, against 20 g per kg of dry matter for concentrates. Increasing the amount of concentrates in dairy cow diets, therefore, would result in a substantial reduction of CH_4 emissions. Implementation of this in practice will lead to an increase in costs associated with the purchase of concentrates, as well as with the problems in setting aside of grassland. Also, the increasing import of 'alien' nutrients from other parts of the world in the farming system will result in increased nutrient surpluses on farm scale or in high costs for nutrient export in animal manure from the farm.
Other diet related options for CH_4 reduction are the use of additives like propionate precursors or probiotics. They are effective in theory, but consumer concern, legislation and limited knowledge limit their applicability in practice.

Housing systems

In table 2, an overview is presented a large survey into the CH_4 emissions from various types of animal housing systems in the Netherlands (Groot Koerkamp & Uenk, 1997). The data show that the amount of CH_4 produced in cow houses is much greater than in pig and poultry houses. However, expressed per kg of live weight (LW), emissions from cattle and pig houses are in the same order of magnitude (0.07–0.16 kg/year per kg of LW), and substantially lower than for poultry (around 0.03 kg/year per kg of LW). Mitigation options for animal housing systems for cattle and pigs are, therefore, equally relevant, and poultry housing related measures will have secondary priority.

Table 2. Methane emissions from Dutch animal housing systems, per animal and per kg of live weight.

Animal type/housing system	Measured methane emission (kg per animal per year)	Assumed average live weight (kg per animal)	Methane emission (kg per year per kg of live weight)
Dairy cows, tie stall	43.9	600	0.07
Dairy cows, cubicles	96.7	600	0.16
Beef cattle, slats	53.8	500	0.11
Veal calves, slats/pens	8.8	100	0.09
Sows, boxes	21.1	200	0.11
Weaners, partly slats	3.9	20	0.15
Fatteners, partly slats	11.1	75	0.15
Laying hens, free range	0.06	2	0.03
Laying hens, cages	0.06	2	0.03
Broilers, litter	0.02	2	0.01

To further assess the potential reduction options for CH_4 from animal housing systems, detailing of the origin of CH_4 needs to be made. Monteny et al. (2001) found that, in general, the CH_4 production ratio from a cow (digestion system) and her manure is 4:1. This implies that dietary measures may have to be considered over manure management options. For pigs, with a less large CH_4 production from the digestion system, this ratio is estimated to be 1:2, whereas CH_4 in poultry husbandry only originate from their excreta. Consequently, manure management will be most effective in reducing CH_4 emissions from pig and poultry houses. Increasing animal productivity, resulting in a reduced number of livestock at an unchanged total production, can also be a way to reduce greenhouse gas emissions, but this solution is not further addressed here.

Adaptation of the housing system is a potential option for greenhouse gas reduction. The data in table 2 show that the CH_4 emission per head from tying stalls for dairy cows is half the emission from dairy cows kept in free stall, cubicle houses. Although the emitting surface area (floor and manure) per cow in tying stalls in much less (around 1 m^2) than in cubicle houses (approximately 3.5 m^2; Monteny & Erisman, 1998), the reducing effect is most likely related to differences in manure management. Typical manure management in tying stalls is the separate collection and storage of feces and urine (with less CH_4 production; see next sub-section), whereas the mixture of feces and urine are stored as slurry under the slatted floor in cubicle houses.

Also for other animal species, changing the housing system will have little effect on the emission greenhouse gases. Besides, this option is in general very costly. On the other hand, improved housing systems from the point of view of e.g. animal welfare or NH_3 emission abatement, may show to have negative side effects in terms of excessive greenhouse gas production. Groenestein & Huis in 't Veld (1994) , and Groenestein & Reitsma (1993) reported CH_4 emissions of around 800 and 1200 g/day and animal for suckling cows and dairy cows, respectively, that were kept in a free range bedding system with straw. This is substantially higher than average CH_4 emissions from cubicle dairy cow housing (500 g; Huis in 't Veld & Monteny, 2003), and can be explained from a contribution of CH_4 from the bedding (microbial decomposition of carbon hydrates) in combination with differences in the diet (mainly in the roughage component). Although no significant emissions of N_2O were reported, Groenestein et al. (1993) reported N_2O emissions of 15-21% of the excreted N in a litter based fattening pig housing system, with introduced micro organisms (to abate NH_3 emissions). These studies clearly indicate that reduction of greenhouse gas emissions from improved animal housing systems may be difficult, and may even enhance those emissions. For straw or litter based systems, negative aspects like the generation of dust has to be considered as well.

Manure management

Manure management is a collection terms for all possibilities that a farmer has to influence the flow or properties of manure on his farm.
One of the most obvious ways for manure management is the direct separation of the solids (faeces) and the liquid (urine). As stated in the previous sub-section, this is conducted in a tying stall, where staw is placed in the gutter behind the animals to collect faeces, and urine is drained separately to a confined storage. Figure 1 shows the results of a laboratory experiment (Monteny, 2003) where CH_4 concentrations from freshly collected dairy cow faeces and manure (slurry) stored in perspex containers (4 L of substrate each) were measured at equal air exchange rates, as a function of temperature. The results show that CH_4 concentrations in the faeces containers are about 50% less when compared to slurry. Also, a clear temperature dependency exists, indicating a temperature related CH_4 production. Direct separation of faeces and urine, however, may not be easy to realize in practice. For dairy cow houses, the so called slit-floor was developed to reduce NH_3 emissions from the pits. Its features enable also separate removal of faeces (by a scraper) and urine (drained throught the holes in the slits to a sub-floor storage).

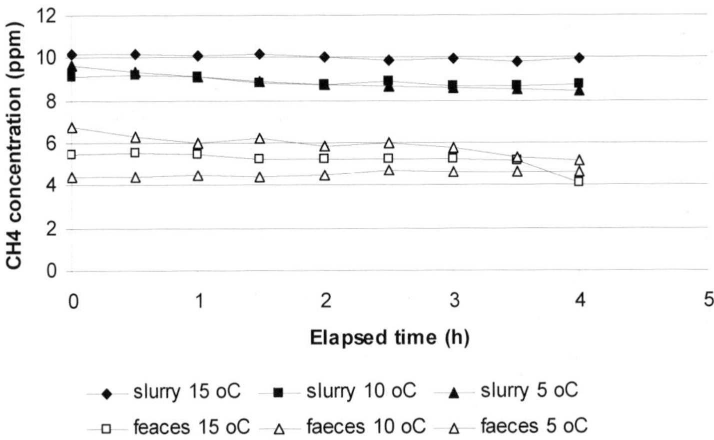

Figure 1. Development of the CH_4 concentration, measured in a laboratory experiment, from freshly collected faeces and slurry from a dairy cow houses as a function of temperature.

Since CH_4 production and temperature are positively related, slurry cooling may also be operated as a slurry management related abatement option. Besides the reduced production, the cooled slurry also reduced the temperature of the air inside the manure pit, thus reducing the air exchange through the slats in the floor (Monteny, 2000).

Another manure management option is minimizing the time that the manure is inside the house. Manure removal should be operated frequently and completely, to avoid or minimize contact between 'old' (inoculation) and 'fresh' manure. Zeeman (1991) clearly demonstrated that CH_4 production is delayed at low inoculation. Types of housing systems that comply with this theory are implemented in practice mainly on pig farms, aiming to reduce NH_3 emissions from the house. They may also benefit CH_4 abatement, under the condition that the removed manure is stored in a confined, covered storage facility outdoors.

Manure treatment

Treatment of manure is defined as the use of additional, specific technology to change the properties of the manure, e.g. aiming at a reduction of gas emissions. A dramatic change in the composition of manure is achieved by the use of manure additives. Berg (1998) investigated the use of lactic acid. They reported significant reductions in NH_3 emissions, due to the lower pH of the manure. Methane emissions were reduced by 50-90%, both for the cow house and indoor storage considered, and for the total farm. This large effect may have been caused by the slowing down of CH_4 production processes, like the breaking down of volatile fatty acids.

Composting is a method for manure treatment that is conducted on farms that produce Farm Yard Manure (FYM), being a mixture of bedding material and manure. Natural composting may occur both inside (in systems with straw bedding or litter) and outside (e.g. dung or FYM heaps). Enforced composing as a way to treat manure, where a focus should be on the forced aeration and moisture content of the substrate. Hüther et al (1997) reported a reduction of CH_4 and N_2O emissions from enforced composting of FYM from cattle and pigs at increasing content of total solids and aeration rates. Both factors will enhance O_2 penetration and distribution and, consequently, result in a more complete oxidation of organic matter to CO_2 and of NH_3 to nitrate (NO_3^-; see equation 1). It has to be noted that this NO_3^- may be de-nitrified at lower aeration conditions, leading to the production of N_2O (equation 2).

Besides aerobic treatment, anaerobic digestion is considered a high potential option to reduce CH_4 emissions. This process, resulting in the controlled production of biogas (mixture of CH_4 and CO_2), is described in detail by Zeeman (1991). A great variation in biogas production of 0 to 1.4 g C per m^3 and h^{-1} is reported (Hansen et al., 2002), depending on the factors indicated previously. From a climate change point of view, this measure is only effective when the biogas produced is used as an energy source, thus replacing non-renewable energy carriers. The feasibility for application in a central (processing plant) or de-central (farm scale) greatly depends on the price of energy and logistic aspects. In any case, the digestate is still considered as animal manure with similar or slightly better N fertilisation properties (increase of NH_3 content from degradation of organic N) than the fresh manure. Other benefits, like the reduction of odour and killing of pathogens, may not contribute to the economic feasibility, but may show to be crucial in the social acceptability of anaerobic digestion.

Pasture management

Nitrous oxide, as a result of nitrification/de-nitrification (equations 1 and 2), is produced upon N excretion in urine (urine patches) by grazing animals and following the application of chemical fertilizers and animal manure. Nitrogen in the manure deposited during grazing, mainly being in the form of urea, is converted to NH_3 by enzymatic urea conversion. The enzyme urease is abundantly available in the faeces and the soil. Velthof et al. (1996, 1997) reported that 1.5-10% (or 10-40 kg N/year and ha) of the N excreted during grazing is lost as N_2O, depending on the soil type. In mechanically applied manure, originating from the house of the outdoor storage, most of the nitrogen is in the form of organic and mineral (NH_3 and NH_4^+). Nitrous oxide emissions after fertilization of grassland are in the same order of magnitude as for grazing (Eichner, 1990; Velthof et al., 1997), where the higher values are found for sandy soils and wet conditions (rain). Moreover, animal manures tend to result in lower N_2O emissions when compared to chemical fertilizers and innovative manure application techniques – like sod injection – may enhance N_2O production and emission. Pasture management may result in a reduced emission of N_2O, when the amount and timing of the applied fertilizers and manure is in harmony with crop demands. This is hardly feasible for grazing, since the dunging and urination behavior of the animals cannot be influenced. Restricted grazing, however, has shown to be effective (Oenema et al., 1997), with an estimated reduction potential of 25% compared to permanent grazing. Negative impacts, like increasing pollutant emissions (mainly NH_3) from the combined housing and grazing, and animal welfare considerations have to be accounted for in the evaluation of the perspectives of restricted grazing. Another option to reduce N_2O from pastures is to optimize the cutting and harvest of grass, thus reducing the amount of crop residues that are left in the field. Also, limitations to grassland renewal has to be considered carefully, not only from and N_2O emission, but also from a NO_3^- leaching point of view. Finally, ground water level adjustment and the introduction of N fixing crops like clover are potential options. Ground water level management can, however, lead to increased CH_4 emissions, especially on peat soils.

Air purification

Air purification is to be considered an ultimate way of removal of harmful gases before the enter the atmosphere. Biofilters, air scubbers and chemical scrubbers are well known for the efficiency in removal of NH_3 and odours from exhaust air. Their penetration in animal husbandry has been low, due to high investment and operational costs, problems with the discharge of waste streams (washing water, salty solution) and additional energy costs for air flow through the purification units.
A recent study by Melse (2003) has shown that a compact biofilter, used for treatment of air from covered storages for liquid manure, is a very effective way to remove not only NH_3 and odour but also to remove CH_4 from this air. The economic aspects and endurance of the unit are still under survey.

Interactions

Losses of NH_3 and N_2O are related to the N cycle on farm scale. Ammonia may emit in all elements of the farming process, whereas N_2O is mainly released as a consequence of N fertilization and grazing. Methane is not directly related to nutrient cycles, since it originates from carbon sources. Brink et al. (2001) concluded that NH_3 emission reducing measures, like new systems for animal housing and manure applications, can also result in increased N_2O emissions mainly from grassland, whereas reduced NH_3 emission and deposition will lower N_2O emissions from natural areas. Moreover, CH_4 emissions were hardly reduced upon the introduction of NH_3 emission abatement strategies. This illustrates the importance of integration of strategies over sources and pollutant emissions and offers a challenge to agricultural, chemical and physical engineers to design integrated solutions against reasonable costs.

Conclusions

Animal husbandry contributes to the emission of the non-CO_2 greenhouse gases methane and nitrous oxide, representing 20% and 35% of the global emissions, respectively. These emissions play a role in the so-called greenhouse effect, represented by global warming and associated problems like depletion of stratospheric ozone.

In-depth knowledge of the processes and influencing factors is essential in the understanding of emission levels and emission inventories, as well as in the design and use of mitigation options. A source approach for methane may be effective, since diet manipulation (e.g. replacement of roughage by concentrates) is a high potential reduction option. For nitrous oxide, the timing and application rate of chemical fertilizers and animal manure have to be adjusted to the crop demand, and minimization of uncontrollable sources like crop residues or manure deposited during grazing can be effective. Yet, drawbacks like applicability and animal welfare have to be considered carefully. Housing systems are hardly effective, and may even show to increase emissions, especially when straw or litter is introduced. Manure management should focus on separation of faeces and urine, or on minimal contact between the manure and the air above. These indoor options are effective when conducted in combination with covered outdoor storage or biogas production. Purification of air from houses and storages has shown to be effective. For all measures, the interaction between technology, management and economy has to be addressed to judge the acceptability in practice. Measures that are already taken in the framework of other gas emissions (e.g. NH_3 emission) are preferable from an integration point of view.

References

Berg, W., 1998. Emissions from animal husbandry and their assessment. Proceedings of the 13th CIGR International Congress on Agricultural Engineering, Rabat, Morocco, February 2-6, p. 289-295.

Brink, C., E.C. Van Ierland, L. Hordijk & C. Kroeze, 2001. Cost-effective emission abatement in Europe considering interrelations in agriculture. In: Optimizing Nitrogen Management in Food and Energy Production and Environmental Protection: Proceedings of the 2nd International Nitrogen Conference on Science and Policy. The Scientific World 1.

Eichner, J.E., 1990. Nitrous oxide emissions from fertilized soils: summary of available data. Journal of Environmental Quality 19: 272-280.

Groenestein, C.M. & B. Reitsma, 1993. Practical research into the ammonia emissions from animal houses X: straw bed house for dairy cattle (In Dutch). Directorate for Agricultural Research (DLO), Report 93-1005, Wageningen, 15 pp. (excl. Annex)

Groenestein, C.M., J. Oosthoek & H.G. Van Faassen, 1993. Microbial processes in deep-litter systems for fattening pigs and emission of ammonia, nitrous oxide and nitric oxide. In: Nitrogen Flow in Pig Production and Environmental Consequences. Proceedings of the First International Symposium, M.W.A.Verstegen, L.A. Den Hartog, G.J.M. Van Kempen & J.H.M. Metz (editors), Pudoc Scientific Publishers, Wageningen, pp. 307 – 312.

Groenestein, C.M. & J.W.H. Huis in 't Veld, 1994. Practical research into the ammonia emissions from animal houses XV: straw bed house for suckling cows (In Dutch). Directorate for Agricultural Research (DLO), Report 94-1006, Wageningen, 14 pp. (excl. Annex)

Groenestein, C.M. & H.G. Van Faassen, 1996. Volatilization of Ammonia, Nitrous Oxide and Nitric Oxide in Deep-litter Systems for Fattening Pigs. Journal of Agricultural Engineering Research 65, 269-274

Groot Koerkamp, P.W.G & G.H. Uenk, 1997. Climatic conditions and aerial pollutants in and emissions from commercial production systems in the Netherlands. In: Ammonia and odour control from animal production facilities. Proceedings of the International Symposium, J.A.M. Voermans & G.J. Monteny (editors), Research Station for Pig Husbandry (PV), Rosmalen, pp. 139 - 144

Hansen, M.N., S.G. Sommer & K. Henriksen, 2002. Methane emissions from livestock manure – effect of storage conditions and climate. In: DIAS-report – Plant Production No. 81. Greenhouse gas inventories for agriculture in Nordic countries, S.O. Pedersen & J.E. Olesen (editors), DIAS, Denmark, p. 45-53.

Houghton, J.T., L.G. Meira Filho, B.A. Callander, N. Harris, A, Kattenberg & K. Maskell, 1996. Climate Change 1995. The Science of Climate Change. Intergovernmental Panel on Climate Change, Cambridge University Press, UK

Huis in 't Veld, J.W.H. & G.J. Monteny, 2003. Methane emissions from cubicle houses for dairy cows (In Dutch). Report 2003-01, Institute of Agricultural and Environmental Engineering, Wageningen, the Netherlands, 27 pp.

Hüther, L., F. Schuchardt & T. Willke, 1997. Emissions of ammonia and greenhouse gases during storage and composting of animal manures. In: Ammonia and odour control from animal production facilities. Proceedings of the International Symposium, J.A.M. Voermans & G.J. Monteny (editors), Research Station for Pig Husbandry (PV), Rosmalen, p. 327 - 334.

Kroeze, C., A. Mosier & L. Bouwman, 1999. Closing the global N_2O budget: a retrospective analysis 1500-1994. Global Biogeochemical Cycles 13 (1): 1-8

Melse, R.W., 2003 Removal of methane from air from a covered liquid manure storage using a pilot-scale biofilter (In Dutch). Institute for Agricultural and Environmental Engineering, IMAG, Nota P 2003-20, Wageningen, the Netherlands.

Monteny, G.J., 2000. Modelling of ammonia emissions from dairy cow houses. PhD Thesis, Wageningen University, Wageningen, the Netherlands, 156 pp.

Monteny, G.J. 2003. Emissions of methane and ammonia from faeces and slurry before and after urine deposition (in progress).

Monteny, G.J. & J.W. Erisman, 1998. Ammonia emissions from dairy cow buildings: a review of measurement techniques, influencing factors and possibilities for reduction. Netherlands Journal of Agricultural Science 46: 225-247.

Monteny, G.J., C.M. Groenestein & M.A. Hilhorst, 2001. Interactions and coupling between emissions of methane and nitrous oxide from animal husbandry. Nutrient Cycling in Agroecosystems 60: 123-132.

Nolan, J.V., 1999. Stoichiometry of rumen fermentation and gas production. In: Meeting the Kyoto Target – Implications for the Australian Livestock Industries, Proceedings of the Workshop, Bureau of Rural Sciences, P.J. Ryenga, & S.M. Howden, Canberra, Australia, pp. 32-40.

Olivier, J.G.J., A.F. Bouwman, K.W. Van der Hoek & J.J.M. Berdowski, 1998. Global air emissions inventories for anthropogenic sources of NO_x, NH_3 and N_2O in 1990. In: Nitrogen, the Confer-N-s. First International Nitrogen Conference, K.W. Van der Hoek et al. (editors), Elsevier, Amsterdam, pp. 135-148.

Veen, W.A.G., 2001. Dietary measures to reduce methane production by ruminants (In Dutch). Institute for Animal Nutrition "De Schothorst", Lelystad, 56 pp.

Velthof, G.L., A.B. Grader & O. Oenema, 1996. Seasonal variation in nitrous oxide losses from managed grassland in the Netherlands. Plant and Soil 181: 263-274.

Velthof, G.L., O. Oenema, R. Postma & M.L. Van Beusichem, 1997. Effects of type and amount of applied nitrogen fertilizer on nitrous oxide fluxes from intensively managed grassland. Nutrient Cycle in Agroecosystems 46: 257-267.

Zeeman, G., 1991. Mesophilic and psychrophilic digestion of liquid manure. PhD Thesis, Wageningen Agricultural University, the Netherlads, 116 pp.

The effects of high ambient temperature on certain physiological parameters on rabbits in Greece

G. Antonakos[1*], E. Xylouri[1], G. Frangiadakis[2], D. Kalogiannis[1] & I. Menegatos[1]
[1]*Agricultural University of Athens, Faculty of Animal Science, Dep of Anatomy and Physiology of Farm Animals, 75, Iera Odos, 118 55, Athens, Greece;* [2]*Dept. of Nutrition and Dietetics, School of Food & Nutrition Technology, Superior, Technological-Education Institute (ATEI) of Crete, Ioannou Kondylaki Street, No 46, 723 00 Siteia, Siteia, Crete, Greece. efxil@aua.gr*

Introduction

The aim of the study was to evaluate the effect of high ambient temperatures on certain male rabbit physiological parameters such as: ALB, AST, ALT, CRP, Ca, Mg, K, Na, Fe, T4 and testosterone.

Materials and methods

Twenty New Zealand bucks were used in two groups of ten. The first group was kept under natural conditions and the second was under temperature-controlled conditions. Blood samples were collected from every buck once a week for three weeks at the time period from the end of July to the beginning of August 2002.

Results and discussion

It is shown that high ambient temperatures alter the biosynthetic capability of liver affecting the concentration of plasma proteins. It also reduces the concentration of hormones, which affect the protein metabolism.

Table 1. Rabbit physiological serum parameters.

physiological parameters	natural conditions[1]	controled conditions[2]	SE	P-value
CRP (mg/dl)	0,82	0,44	0.12	0.0300
ALT (u/1)	28,60	045.50	2,59	0.0000
Mg (mg/dl)	2.13	2,937	0,08	0.0000
Fe (ug/dl)	117,60	156.45	6,99	0.0002
T4 (nmol/1)	36,46	41.23	1,57	0.0360
Testosterone (ng/ml)	3.24	4,97	0.55	0.0290
CRP/ALB	251.39	120.05	42.18	0.0317
CRP/ALT (mg/U)	0.37	0.13	0.065	0.0111

[1]28.5 °C, [2]25.6 °C,

Conclusions

Proper modification of the nutrition seems to be able to alleviate the negative effects of thermal stress on bucks.

References

Marai I.F.M. et al., 2002. Livestock Prod. Sci. 78:71-90.
Boiti C. et al., 1992. J. Appl. Rabbit Res. 15:447-455.

Oxidative status in transition dairy cows under heat stress conditions

U. Bernabucci*, N. Lacetera, A. Nardone & B. Ronchi
Dipartimento di Produzioni Animali, Università della Tuscia, 01100 Viterbo, Italy. bernab@unitus.it

Introduction

Alteration of OxS in periparturient HSed dairy cows (Bernabucci et al., 2002) and in obese periparturient dairy cows (Ronchi et al., 2000) have been reported. Little is known in ruminants about the relationships between oxidative status (OxS) and metabolic status in transition heat-stressed (HSed) dairy cows.

Materials and methods

Three weeks before calving 12 Holstein heifers were divided in two groups and housed in two climatic chambers until 50 days in milk. One group (HTHI) was exposed to high temperature-humidity index (THI) conditions (82 THI from 09.00 to 20.00 h; 76 THI from 21.00 to 08.00 h), the other one (TC) was exposed to thermal-comfort conditions (68 THI for 24 hours). Feed (DMI) and water consumption were measured daily. Rectal temperatures (RT) and respiration rates (RR) were recorded weekly. Every two weeks blood samples were taken from the jugular vein. On plasma samples glucose, nonesterified fatty acids (NEFA), β-OH-butyrate (BHBA), reactive oxygen metabolites (ROMs), thiol groups (SHp) and malondialdehyde (MDA) were determined. Data were analysed as repeated measures using the GLM procedure of SAS®. Correlation among parameters were determined. Significance were declared at $P<0.05$.

Results and discussion

HTHI heifers had higher ($P<0.05$) RT and RR (39.5 vs. 38.8°C and 70 vs. 43 breaths/min, respectively), lower DMI (-20%) and milk yield (17.1 vs. 21.4 litre/d of 4% FCM). HTHI heifers had more severe energy deficit with higher ($P<0.05$) plasma NEFA and BHBA and lower ($P<0.05$) plasma glucose before and after calving compared with TC. MDA picked two weeks postpartum and was higher in HTHI compared with TC. ROMs were higher before calving and lower in early lactation in HTHI compared with TC. SHp were not affected by treatment, and showed higher values around calving (Table 1).

Table 1. Changes of plasma marker of oxidative status (a,b = $P < 0.05$).

		Days from calving						
		-15	-3	1	13	20	34	48
ROMs, mgH_2O_2/100 ml	HTHI	15.3 [b]	16.9 [b]	17.4 [b]	16.7 [a]	13.8 [a]	14.6	10.6
	TC	11.7 [a]	12.8 [a]	14.5 [a]	19.1 [b]	17.3 [b]	16.0	13.2
SHp, µmol/L	HTHI	216.2	221.9	227.0	190.0	150.0	71.0	101.1
	TC	203.0	222.3	235.1	175.7	151.2	131.1	115.7
MDA, µmol/L	HTHI	19.8	30.6 [b]	38.0	105.0 [b]	47.2	26.1	33.5
	TC	28.7	10.3 [a]	26.0	86.7 [a]	44.9	40.0	33.0

Significant relationships ($P<0.05$) were found between ROMs and MDA (r=0.42), ROMs and BHBA (r=0.46), MDA and NEFA (r=0.49), and MDA and glucose (r= -0.47) under HTHI. Under hot environment periparturient dairy cows present some variation of the oxidative status, and the oxidative damages are more likely in cows exhibiting the more severe energy deficit.

Conclusions

Risk of oxidative stress is increased by exposure to HTHI. The study revealed the existence of relationships between the oxidative status and metabolic-nutritional conditions in periparturient HSed dairy cows.

References

Bernabucci U. et al., 2002. J. Dairy Sci. 85:2173-2179.
Ronchi B. et al., 2000. 51st Annual Meeting EAAP, 212.

The effect of climatic conditions on performances of dairy cows in Tunisia

R. Bouraoui[1*], M. Lahmar[2], A. Majdoub[3] & M. Djemali[3]
[1]Ecole Supérieure d'Agriculture de Mateur, 7030 Mateur, Tunisia, [2]Institut National de la Recherche Agronomique de Tunisie, 2049 Ariana, Tunisia, [3]Institut National Agronomique de Tunisie, 1082 Tunis, Tunisia. bouraoui@iresa.agrinet.tn

Introduction

The objective of the present work is to identify thermal stress areas in Tunisia and to determine the effect of heat stress on performances of lactating Friesian-Holstein cows using the Temperature Humidity Index (THI) developed in the United states by Johnson.

Materials and methods

In a first step, a ten-year period weather data obtained from 24 weather stations located all over the country were used to calculate the THI and to subsequently establish seasonal heat stress maps. In a second step, 4 different geographical locations in north and central Tunisia were selected to investigate the relationship between heat stress and performances of cows. For each herd in these locations, milk production data for a 10-year period and reproduction data for 7 years were analysed for these locations, and relationships between milk yield, reproduction parameters and THI values were established.

Results and discussion

Results showed that Tunisia is under heat stress between June and September with THI values ranging between 72 and 78, except for the regions of Tozeur and Kebili in the south which are characterized by THI values over 78. The summer and the fall seasons showed the highest THI values and were unfavourable to maximum production of exotic dairy breeds In fact, lactation peaks were 22.7; 22.8; 21.3 and 21.4 kg per cow per day for the winter, the spring, the fall and the summer, respectively. Overall milk production per cow showed a 10% drop between the months of March and September going from 17.1 to 15.3 kg, respectively. In addition, milk composition data indicated that milk fat content differed slightly between summer and winter (3.69 Vs 3.80 %). First conception rate (TRI_1) and overall conception rate (CR) were lowest in the summer for the four experimental sites (25 and 32 % for TRI_1 and CR respectively for the month of August). The highest values (58.9 for TRI_1 and 51 % for CR) were observed for the month of February. Regression equations between THI and TRI_1 and THI and CR showed high R^2 values of 0.70 and 0.89 respectively, suggesting an important relationship between heat stress and these indicators. Calving and Calving-conception intervals were the longest for cows calving between May and July and the shortest for those calving between December and January.

Conclusions

It was concluded that climatic conditions, as expressed in term of THI, affected milk production and reproductive efficiency of dairy cows in Tunisia.

Factors affecting some blood parameters and rectal temperature in cows in the Tropics

F. Cerutti, R. Rizzi*, M. Faustini & C. Colombani
Dipartimento di Scienze e Tecnologie Veterinarie per la Sicurezza Alimentare, Università degli Studi, 20133 Milano, Via Celoria 10, Italy. rita.rizzi@unimi.it

Introduction

Under heat stress condition the ability of a cow to maintain the energetic, mineral and thermal balance is a good indicator of adaptability to environment. The present study was carried on cows in the Tropics and the objective in the first phase was to study the environmental factors as possible source of the variability of blood parameters and rectal temperature.

Materials and methods

The study included 400 cows (straightbred Holstein and Carora; and ½ Carora ½ Holstein, ¼ Carora ¾ Holstein, ½ Carora ½ Zebu crosses) in 4 herds of Venezuela from February 2000 to June 2001. Blood samples were collected 15 days before calving, at 45 and at 90 days after calving by vacum glass tubes without anticoagulant. Serum analyses were performed by an automated analyzer for total proteins, cholesterol, triglycerides, urea, alanine aminotransferase (ALT), aspartate aminotransferase (AST), calcium, inorganic phosphorus and magnesium. In the drawing days rectal temperature was measured at 0600 h and at 1800 h. Blood parameters and rectal temperature were analyzed by a mixed model including the fixed effects of herd, drawing year-month interaction, breed, age, and drawing day and the random effect of cow within herd.

Results and discussion

The drawing day showed a significant effect on all blood parameters with the exception of minerals. After calving the increase of cholesterol and the decrease of triglycerides were observed. Those changes may be related in part to lactogenesis and milking and to the mammary metabolism of lipoproteins (Guédon et al., 1999). Urea increased after calving in agreement with Ronchi et al. (1998). The year-month of collection significantly affected cholesterol, triglycerides, ALT and AST. In the hottest months the cholesterol and triglycerides level decreased and the liver enzymes increased. In herds under favorable climatic conditions cows showed high cholesterol levels. A slightly significant effect of breed group on cholesterol was found ($0.05<P<0.01$). The lowest cholesterol levels were observed in Holsteins (125 mgl/dl) and in ½ Carora ½ Holstein crosses (119 mg/dl), whereas the highest levels were found in ½ Carora ½ Zebu cows (153 mg/dl). Rectal temperature was significantly influenced by all factors except age. Cows presented higher rectal temperature in the hottest months and at noon. The highest values were found in two herds under unfavorable conditions. However, in the herd with a large number of Holsteins rectal temperature was higher (39.4°C) than in the herd with many Carora cows (39.1°C). Breed groups significantly differed in rectal temperature, the highest value being observed for Holsteins (39.3°C) and the lowest for ½ Carora ½ Holstein crosses (39.0°C).

Conclusions

Cholesterol, ALT, AST and rectal temperature are affected by climatic conditions. Cholesterol levels could be an indicator of heat stress in dairy cows since cholesterolemia decreases as temperature increases. Moreover, an increase in cholesterol was observed in breed groups with a good adaptation to environment and in breed groups and indigenous groups with the lowest rectal temperatures.

References

Guédon L. et al., 1999. Theriogenology 51:1405-1415.
Ronchi B. et al., 1998. Zoot. Nutr. Anim. 24:283-293.

Acknowledgements

Research financed by Cofinanziamento MURST 1999.

Genetic characterisation of Nellore and Criolla cattle: preliminary results

S. Conti[1*], R. Bozzi[1], D. Marletta[2], A. Giorgetti[1] P. Degl'Innocenti[1] & A. Martini[1]
[1]Dipartimento di Scienze Zootecniche, Università di Firenze, [2]Dipartimento di Produzioni Animali, Università di Catania, Italy. sconti@unifi.it

Introduction

Microsatellites are used to assess the genetic diversity among cattle breeds in several studies. We carried out a research project on genetic variability of Nellore and Criolla cattle, two tropical cattle breeds acclimatized to warm climate. This study reports the first results on genetic variability of these breeds.

Materials and methods

Blood samples were collected from 50 unrelated animals of each of the two cattle breeds (Criolla and Nellore). DNA was extracted from fresh blood following the protocol based on Buffer, Ethanol and Proteinase K. The sixteen loci: BM1818, BM1824, BM2113, MM12, HAUT24, HAUT27, ILSTS005, ILSTS006, TGLA227, TGLA126, TGLA122, TGLA53, ETH3, ETH225, ETH10, SPS115 were amplified in five simplex PCR and four multiplex PCR. PCR reaction was carried out on 2 μl of DNA solution in 10.25 μl final volume containing 2.4 μl 10X PCR Buffer (Perkin Elmer), 0.6 μl $MgCl_2$ solution (25mM, Perkin Elmer), 3 μl of the dNTPs solution (10nm each), 2 μl of each primer (10μM), and 0,25 μl of AmpliTaqGold ™ (5U/μl, Perkin Elmer). PCR products were mixed with GeneScan 350 Tamra internal size standard. Polyacrylamide gel electrophoresis and genotype determination were performed on an ABI Prism 311 DNA Sequencer. The GENEPOP (Raymond et al., 1995) and DISPAN (Ota, 1993) packages were used to calculate allelic frequencies, expected and observed heterozigosity, and gene diversity parameters.

Results and discussion

The number of alleles at each locus range from 7 to 16. The highest value was found for the ETH03 locus (0.67) whereas the lowest (0.009) has been found in various loci. The two breeds showed almost the same mean number of alleles. Expected heterozigosity was higher in Nellore breed whereas the observed one was similar between the two populations (Table 1). The value of expected heterozigosity found for Criolla is comparable to that found by Postiglioni et al. (2002) on Uruguayan Criolla population. The gene diversity parameters showed that almost all the diversity (Ht = 0.70) has retained within the breeds and that the gene differentiation between populations is low (Gst = 0.067).

Table 1. Number of alleles frequencies, expected and observed heterozigosity (± s.e.)

Breed	Mean n° of alleles ± s.d.	Exp. Het. ± s.e.	Obs. Het. ± s.e.
Nellore	7.37 ± 2.68	0.73 ± 0.01	0.45 ± 0.02
Criolla	6.81 ± 1.17	0.67 ± 0.01	0.45 ± 0.03

Conclusions

Data obtained in this study indicate that Nellore and Criolla cattle breeds, despite their different population size, showed a genetic variability comparable to those reported for other cattle breeds (Edwards et al., 2000; Martin-Burriel et al., 1999). The gene diversity parameters found here assure that even for the Criolla cattle, threatened of extinction, exists the possibility to select with low risks of reduction of genetic variability.

References

Raymond M. et al., 1995. J. Heredity 86:248-249.
Ota T., 1993. Penn. St. Univ.
Postiglioni A. et al., 2002. Arch. Zootecn. 51:248-249.
Edwards et al., 2000. Anim. Gen. 31:329-332.
Martin-Burriel et al., 1999. Anim. Gen. 30:177-182.

Acknowledgments

Research supported by Cofinanziamento MURST 1999 funds. Responsible Prof. Andrea Martini.

The effect of environmental temperature and humidity on cashmere yield, secondary active follicles and thyroid hormones in cashmere goats

A. Di Trana[1*], P. Celi[1] & R. Celi[2]
[1]Dipartimento di Scienze delle Produzioni Animali, Università della Basilicata, 85100 Potenza, Italy, [2]Dipartimento Pro. Ge. Sa., Università di Bari, 70126 Bari, Italy. ditrana@unibas.it

Introduction

Little is known on effects of environmental temperature and humidity on cashmere yield and hair follicle activity. Thyroid hormones levels is influenced by ambient temperature and their concentrations seem to affect hair follicles activity. The aim of this study was to evaluate changes of cashmere yield (CY), secondary active follicles (SAF) and circulating triiodothyronine (T_3) and thyroxine (T_4) in cashmere bearing goats kept under different Temperature Humidity Index (THI).

Materials and methods

Two groups of ten cashmere goats each, homogeneous for live weight and age were used. Cashmere yield measured in the previous cycle was similar in the two groups. During the months June–April, one group was maintained in a site characterized by Low THI (L) and the other group, six months before the beginning of the trial, was moved in a site characterized by High THI (H). Goats were kept on native pastures, supplemented with 200g concentrate and hay *ad libitum*. Every two months, we measured THI, CY, SAF as described by Di Trana et al. (2001). Plasma concentration of T_3 and T_4 were assayed by RIA. Data were analysed using ANOVA for repeated measures.

Results and discussion

Results are summarized in Table 1. CY was higher in the goats kept at L in August and December. Similarly, more SAF were found in goats at L site in August and October as previously observed by Celi et al. (2002). Plasma T_3 concentrations were affected by THI and time. T_4 levels were significantly affected by time ($P<0.05$) but not by THI. The finding that both CY and SFA were higher in L suggest that locations characterized by low THI are more suitable for cashmere yield. In this study T_3 levels were higher in goats kept at L than H during the period in which cashmere growth occurs. Considering that high levels of thyroid hormones have been related to active fibre growth (Rhind et al., 1995) our data support a positive role of thyroid hormones in follicle activity.

Table 1. Mean values of cashmere yield, secondary active follicles, T_3 and T_4 concentration in cashmere goats reared at sites with low and high Temperature Humidity Index.

Month	THI		CY %		SAF %		T_3 ng/dl		T_4 µg/dl	
	L	H	L	H	L	H	L	H	L	H
June	70	76	0.0	0.0	37.9	25.1	137.91	149.15	3.34	3.75
August	74	79	15.4a	4.6b	74.2a	51.9b	107.27	100.34	3.65	3.62
October	62	68	27.3	20.6	84.9A	60.3B	113.89a	84.02b	3.26	3.09
December	51	58	38.0a	30.1b	68.0	75.7	90.38	104.91	3.64	4.27
February	49	57	35.0	30.0	35.8	27.0	104.70	123.55	3.96	4.43
April	57	64	14.6	22.5	24.5	18.1	95.44B	164.09A	3.12	4.12
Pooled SE			3.6		7.7		12.19		0.42	

A, B: P<0.01; a, b: P<0.05 within the same row

Conclusions

Our results indicate that different sites with low THI favour CY, SAF. T_3 seem to promote secondary hair follicle activity and cashmere yield.

References

Celi P. et al., 2002. Ital. J. Anim. Sci. 1:79-86.
Di Trana A. et al., 2001. Proc.14th Congr. ASPA 526-528.
Rhind S.M. et al., 1995. Small Ruminant Res. 16:69-76.

Acknowledgements

The study was financially supported by MURST Cofin.-1999.

Ultrastructural characterization of rabbit sperm abnormalities under heat stress conditions

A.M. Fausto[1]*, A.R. Taddei[2], G. Kuzminsky[3] & P. Morera[3]
[1]Dipartimento di Scienze Ambientali, [2]Centro Interdipartimentale di Microscopia Elettronica, [3]Dipartimento di Produzioni Animali, Università della Tuscia, 01100 Viterbo, Italy. fausto@unitus.it

Introduction
Reduced reproductive efficiency in male rabbits is commonly observed during summer months in tropical and subtropical countries. A previous study (Finzi et al., 1995) showed that morphological abnormalities of spermatozoa increased in number in condition of chronic heat stress, suggesting that this parameter could have been used to test both sperm quality and breeding conditions with reference to high ambient temperature (HAT). In the present work, ultrastructural abnormalities of rabbits spermatozoa, have been characterised and their relative frequencies in both pre-stress and stress period, have been investigated in order to verify the influence of HAT on sperm morphology.

Materials and methods
Ten male N.Z.W. rabbits at the same age (9 months), body weight (Kg 4.0 ± 0.2), and sperm output were placed in a climatic chamber at 20°C and relative humidity at 70% for an adaptation period of three weeks. The animals were then kept at ambient temperatures of 29.8°C ± 0.6 for 22 hours a day and 24.7°C ± 0.8 for 2 hours a day for 9 weeks. Ejaculated spermatozoa were collected by artificial vagina. Sperm abnormalities were studied by scanning (SEM) and transmission (TEM) electron microscopy. The sperm were processed as previously reported (Kuzminsky et al 1996 ; Fausto et al. 2001).

Results and discussion
SEM and TEM analyses of the spermatozoa collected in both pre-stress and stress periods showed the same morphological abnormalities. Some of these have been sporadically observable, while others have been always present in all specimens. In many cases, the same type of abnormalities can be described at both SEM and TEM levels. However, TEM analyses also evidenced abnormalities that haven't involved the external morphology of the cell and haven't been detectable by SEM. The morphological abnormalities were grouped in three types: head and tail abnormalities and sperm in degeneration (teratoid spermatozoa). We found head abnormalities in shape and size, acrosome (knobbed, vesiculated, absent acrosome), nuclear vacuoles and abnormal DNA condensation. The most frequent tail abnormalities were: tails with proximal or distal cytoplasmic droplets, bent tails, coiled tails, multiple tails axonemal and mitochondrial abnormalities. Quantitative analyses of the spermatozoa, collected in both pre-stress and stress periods, showed a significant increase of total morphological abnormalities from the first week of heat stress period (25% vs 39%, + 56%, P< 0.05). The reached peak at the fourth week of heat stress (25% vs 43%, +72%, P< 0.01) was followed by decreasing values that at ninth week were still higher in comparison with the control period (25% vs 36%, + 44%, P<0.05).

Conclusions
Rabbit sperm were found to be very sensitive to HAT because it showed changes in the percentages of morphological abnormalities. These abnormalities, ultrastructurally described, could affect fertility as reported in other species (Barth et al., 1989).

References
Finzi A. et al., 1995. World Rabbit Sci. 3:157-161.
Kuzminsky G. et al., 1996. Reprod. Nutr. Dev. 36:565-575.
Fausto A.M. et al., 2001. Reprod. Nutr. Dev., 41:217-225.
Barth A.D. et al., 1989. Abnormal Morphology of Bovine Spermatozoa, 1st ed.University Press, Ames, IO, USA, 1:285.

Categorizing heat load in grain-fed beef cattle – New approaches

J.B. Gaughan[1*] & R.A. Eigenberg[2]
[1]*School of Animal Studies, The University of Queensland, Gatton, Queensland, 4343 Australia,* [2]*US Meat Animal Research Center, Clay Center, Nebraska, 68933 USA. jbg@sas.uq.edu.au*

Introduction
The traditional approach to heat stress in cattle has been to categorize the severity of the stress by using environmental measures, such as, the temperature humidity index (THI). However, THI does not take into account impact of solar load or wind. Furthermore, the best indicator of the severity of the heat load, the animal, is not included. To overcome this, new indices, the heat load index (HLI) and estimated respiration rate (EstRR) incorporating animal behaviour, ambient temperature (Ta), relative humidity (RH,%), wind speed (WS, m/s) and solar radiation (SR, w/m^2) have been developed by Gaughan (HLI) and Eigenberg (EstRR) respectively.

Materials and methods
For the development of the HLI long-fed Angus steers (n = 2490) from four Australian feedlots were used in a 102 day study over the 2002 Australian summer. Two shaded and two unshaded pens were used at each feedlot. In the development of EstRR eight *Bos taurus* steers were used. At any one time four steers (in individual pens) had access to shade and four did not. The cattle were moved eight times so that each animal had access to shade or no shade four times (8 days periods). In the first study location in pen e.g. at water trough, and activity e.g. standing or lying were recorded. In both studies DMI, panting scores (PS) and respiration rate (RR) were recorded. A five point (0, 1, 2, 3, 4) score was used with PS 0 being normal and PS 4 being extreme distress – RR>160 breaths/min (bpm), open mouth, tongue out, drooling and head down. Body temperature was collected in study 2. In both studies Ta, RH, WS, SR, and black globe temperature (BGT, °C) were collected. Regression analysis was used to determine the relative importance of the measured weather data on cattle behaviour and physiology.

Results and discussion
HLI and EstRR provide numerical values which can be used to categorise the level of "stress" (Table 1). WS had a major impact on HLI. At a given Ta and RH were WS = 0, HLI had a higher value than THI. However, HLI decreased almost linearly as WS increased from 0 to 3 m/s, the effect then plateaued. Four heat load categories have been defined based on animal observation and physiological response. The categories are for unshaded *Bos taurus* cattle exposed to Ta>25°C, and are for the average animal. Under any given HLI or EstRR individuals may be experiencing more or less heat load. It is crucial that cattle are observed during Danger and Emergency on a regular basis e.g. every 2 hours. The time of day is also an important consideration. A Danger category at 1800 h when conditions are cooling off is not as critical as an Alert at 0600 h going into a potentially hot day

Table 1. Heat load index (HLI) and EstRR, category and description

HLI	EstRR	Category	Description for Unshaded Cattle
<79	<85 bpm	Normal	No heat load problems
79 - 84	85 - 110	Alert	Mild heat load effects especially on vulnerable cattle
84 - 90	110 - 133	Danger	Strong to severe heat load effects on cattle
91 +	>133	Emergency	Severe to extreme effects on cattle – death possible

Conclusion
The HLI and EstRR are suitable indicators of heat load status of grain fed *Bos taurus* cattle. The indices are currently being assessed under field conditions.

Using panting scores to assess heat load in cattle

J.B. Gaughan
School of Animal Studies, The University of Queensland, Gatton, Queensland, 4343 Australia. jbg@sas.uq.edu.au

Introduction

Respiration rate (RR) and panting scores (PS) are useful indicators of heat load in cattle because an increase is often the first visual response to hot conditions. Both are primarily influenced by ambient temperature (Ta) and are easy to observe. PS offers additional information on the heat load status of cattle (Table 1). The PS concept was developed by Mader et al. (2001), and a modified by Gaughan et al. (2002). PS range from 0 (normal) to 4.5 (animal severely stressed) (Table 1). Cattle with a PS ≥ 3.5 are in danger and without some form of relief from the hot conditions death is possible.

Table 1. Breathing Condition and Panting Score (PS).

Breathing Condition	PS
No panting – normal.	0
Slight panting, mouth closed, no drool or foam.	1
Fast panting, drool or foam present.	2
As for 2 but with occasional open mouth.	2.5
Open mouth + some drooling. Neck extended and head usually up.	3
As for 3 but with tongue out slightly	3.5
Open mouth tongue out + drooling. Neck extended and head up.	4
As for 4 but head held down.	4.5

Materials and methods

The PS concept was tested at an Australian feedlot on 14 occasions over the Australian summer (December–March). PS were first observed on two cool days THI < 70 in order to establish a base line. On these days all cattle were observed with a PS of 0 (PS0). PS were observed (every hour from 0600 h to 1800 h) for cattle in two shaded and two un-shaded pens. The pen specifications were: 150 head/pen; pen area = 3200 m^2; 22 m^2 /head. The shaded pens had approximately 4 m^2 of shade/head.

Results and discussion

Approximately 50% of cattle in the shaded pen were under the shade between 1100 and 1500 h. Mean maximum Ta and relative humidity on the 12 hot days were 35.7°C and 25.4% respectively. There were significantly greater numbers in the un-shaded pens with PS>0 in comparison to the shaded pens (79.9% vs. 33.1%). Only 0.5% of the shaded cattle had a PS greater than 1 compared to 7.7% for the un-shaded cattle. Typically PS moved from 0 to 1 at approximately 25°C, 1 - 2 at 30°C and were 3 or greater when Ta was greater than 35°C. However, this was also influenced by degree of cloud cover. PS were lower when cloud cover was greater than 50% then when exposed to similar Ta with no clouds. Eating activity did not appear to influence PS.

Conclusions

PS are an effective management tool to assist in the assessment of stress levels due to heat in grain fed cattle, and should be used as part of summer management. During periods of adverse hot weather the PS of vulnerable cattle should be assessed before 0800 h, and then at 2-hour intervals at least until 1800 h. PS has the potential to be used in the assessment of the welfare status of cattle

References

Mader T.L. et al., 2001. In: 2001 Nebraska Beef Cattle Report. University of Nebraska Lincoln NE 119.
Gaughan J.B. et al., 2002. Meat Livestock Australia, Nth. Sydney NSW 56.

Seasonal variations of milk quality in Parmigiano-Reggiano cheese manufacture on a period of 10 years

M. Malacarne[1*], E. Fossa[2], S. Sandri[2], F. Tosi[2], A. Summer[1] & P. Mariani[1]
[1]*Dipartimento di Produzioni Animali BVQSA, Università di Parma, 43100 Parma,* [2]*Centro Lattiero Caseario, 43100 Parma, Italy. massimo.malacarne@unipr.it*

Introduction

In the Parmigiano-Reggiano cheese manufacture, the milk quality payment system consider the following parameters: casein (IR protein x 0.77) and fat content, titratable acidity (TA), somatic cells count (SCC), total bacterial count (TBC), presence of *Clostridia* spores (>100 spores/l) and coliforms (>5000 UFC/ml), lactodynamographic (LDG) type, presence of inhibitors. The physiological, environmental and feeding factors markedly influence milk quality (Ng-Kwai-Hang et al., 1982; Bertoni et al., 2001). Aim of this research was to study the seasonal variations of these parameters on a 10 years period.

Materials and methods

The study was carried out on about 83000 herd milk samples collected monthly from 1991 to 2000. Conditions and time of sampling and methods of analysis were described by Sandri et al., 2001. Presence of inhibitors was not studied. Monthly mean values (120 obs) were analyzed by two way (season, year) ANOVA (SPSS).

Results and discussion

The values of milk quality parameters (table 1) worsen from Winter to Spring, except % of LDG type with low (E) and scarce coagulability (F) (unvaried) and *Clostridia* % positive (improve). In summer most values worsen, except fat content, % of samples with high (e) and very high (ee) level of TBC, both unvaried, and casein content (improve). In Autumn, almost all parameter improve, except *Clostridia* %, which remain unvaried. Besides climatic factors, these variation are also related to the season of calving, mostly in Autumn and Winter, and variation of feeding during the year.

Table 1. Least square mean values of milk quality parameters by season.

		Winter	Spring	Summer	Autumn	Overall	SD
Casein	g/100g	2.36b	2.34a	2.36b	2.46c	2.38	0.07
Fat	g/100g	3.68b	3.54a	3.56a	3.77c	3.64	0.12
TA	°SH/50ml	3.23c	3.20b	3.17a	3.21bc	3.20	0.05
SCC	10^3/ml	313a	345b	400c	350b	351	39
TBC	% e+ee	8.51a	12.76b	12.56b	8.85a	10.50	3.53
Coliforms	% positive	1.98a	6.50c	10.79d	3.03b	4.52	5.74
Cl. spores	% positive	13.18b	12.30a	16.18c	16.11c	14.35	4.76
LDG	% E+F type	18.88a	21.93ab	43.05c	24.89b	25.82	15.26

Values with different letters (a, b, c and d) differ for $P<0.05$

Conclusions

The overall dairy-technological quality of milk register a decrease from Winter to Spring and to Summer, and an improve in Autumn. These results agree with others studies (Bernabucci et al., 1998; Calamari et al., 1998).

References

Bernabucci U. et al., 1998. Zoot. Nutr. Anim. 24:247-257.
Bertoni G. et al., 2001. Proc. Nutr. Soc., 60:231-246.
Calamari L. et al., 1998. Zoot. Nutr. Anim., 24:259-271.
Ng-Kwai-Hang K.F. et al., 1982. J. Dairy Sci., 65:1993-1998.
Sandri S. et al., 2001. Ann. Fac. Med. Parma, 21:235-247 http://www.unipr.it/arpa/facvet/annali/index.htm.

Acknowledgements

This work was supported by CRPA, Reggio Emilia, Italy.

Macrominerals in buffalo at different physiological state during winter and summer

Zia-ur-Rahman, M. Ashraf & A. Khan
Department of Physiology and Pharmacology, University of Agriculture, Faisalabad, Pakistan. drziar@yahoo.com

Introduction

Generally buffalo serve to meet dietary milk, meat and farm work requirements as well as a source of income. Animals receive adequate amounts of minerals in the rainy season than that of dry season (Mpofu, et al., 1999). Minerals level of animal feed and its absorption into the animal in different seasons may help improve nutrition constraints limiting animal productivity and health.Therefore, investigation on bioavailability of macro nutrients in different seasons was executed.

Materials and methods

100g of feed samples were collected from animal ration for its composition and macromineral analysis. Blood, milk, urine and fecal samples were taken from buffalo at different physiological state.All samples were properly stored till further analysis. All samples were digested and macro minerals were estimated by Flamephotometer.

Results and discussion

Na^+ concentration in feed varied significantly during the summer season. Plasma and urine contained significantly lower Na^+ concentration in both lactating and non lactating buffaloes. However, the highest excretion of Na^+ was observed through feces of lactating and non lactating buffaloes. In lactating buffaloes the fecal Na^+ concentration was significantly higher during summer than that in winter, but the reverse was true for non lactating buffaloes. Tiffany et al. (1999) observed that seasonal variation in Na+ forage concentration was observed in year are but there was no consistent pattern. Potassium (K^+) excretion was higher in the urine as well as in feces during summer season. In addition, plasma K^+ level were also significantly higher in non-lactating buffaloes irrespective of season. Cl^- concentration in feed did not vary significantly during each season. Plasma and feces contained significantly lower concentration of Cl^- than those in milk and urine in lactating buffaloes and that in urine in non-lactating buffaloes. The highest excretion of Cl^- was observed through the urine of both lactating and non-lactating buffaloes during both seasons.

Conclusions

It can be concluded that buffaloes were fed feed that is different in minerals composition in winter and summer seasons.

References

Mpofu I.D.T. et al., 1999. Asian. Aust. J. Anim. Sci. 12(4):579-584.
Tiffany M.E. et al., 1999. Commun. Soil Sci. Plant Anal. 30 (19&20):2743-2754.

Microminerals in buffalo at different physiological state during winter and summer

Zia-ur-Rahman, M. Ashraf & A. Khan
Department of Physiology and Pharmacology, University of Agriculture, Faisalabad, Pakistan. drziar@yahoo.com

Introduction

By evaluating the minerals level of animal feed and its absorption into the animal in different reasons may help improve nutrition constraints that limit animal productivity and health condition. Therefore, investigation on bioavailability of micro nutrients in different seasons was determined at a farm and in buffalo.

Materials and methods

Blood samples were taken from buffalo at different physiological state, plasma separated and stored at -4°C. Morning and evening milk samples were collected and KCr_2O_7 was added as preservative. Fecal samples of buffalo were collected in plastic bags twice daily and stored at –20°C for further analysis. Plasma, milk, urine and fecal samples were digested and micro minerals were estimated by Atomic Absorption Photometer.

Results and discussion

Plasma concentration of Mg^{2+} in lactating and non-lactating buffalo did not differ significantly. Mg level of 0.06 to 0.08 mmol/liter are considered to be safe and animals with less than 0.4 mmol/liter are exposed to the risk of disease (McDowell, 1985). Higher plasma Mg^{2+} concentration may be indicative of supply and demand of the animals and excrete more Mg^{2+} through feces than urine. In lactating buffalo, Fe plasma showed a marked excretion through feces during winter season. High fecal Fe levels reflects high consumption of Fe either from the diet. Plasma manganese contents in lactating buffaloes were negligible, despite the fact that animals require more minerals during their lactation period. Plasma manganese contents in non-lactating animals were higher than those of lactating animals, although non-lactating buffaloes excreted higher manganese in their feces than the lactating ones. Urine manganese contents in lactating buffaloes were significant higher than non-lactatings. Plasma Cu^{2+} concentration was significantly lower irrespective of their physiological condition and suggest that buffalo are susceptible to Cu^{2+} deficiencies throughout the years. Cu^{2+} absorption may be influenced by age, some hormones, pregnancy and some diseases (Goodrich et al., 1972). Zn^{2+} in lactating buffaloes tended to be higher in summer season than in winter season. The amount of Zn^{2+} passed through the feces differed highly significantly in lactating and non lactating buffaloes ($P<0.001$) in the two seasons.

Conclusions

It can be concluded that buffalo raised at the farm are fed diet that is different in micro-minerals composition during winter and summer seasons. Threfore, micro-minerals supplementation is suggested to increase productivity in buffalo.

References

Goodrich R.D. et al., 1972. Proc. Minnesota Nutr. Conf. p 169.

McDowell L.R., 1985. In: Nutrition of Grazing Ruminants in Warm Climates, Academic Press, New York. pp 165-188.

A higher susceptibility of hyperthermic animals to infectious disease

Masaaki Shibata
Department of Biometeorology, Yamanashi Institute of Environmental Sciences, Fuji-Yoshida, Yamanashi 403-0005, Japan. mshibata@yies.pref.yamanashi.jp

Introduction
High body temperature (hyperthermia) changes physiological functions that include cardiovascular, endocrine, and body fluid systems. Hyperthermia can produce either detrimental or beneficial effects on animal and human health. This study describes the former case, and addresses mechanisms to explain why animals develop more severe endotoxin fever after they recover from hyperthermia.

Materials and methods
Male rabbits were made transiently hyperthermic by raising their normal body temperature up to 43 °C in a chamber kept at 44 °C. They were then allowed to recover in a room at 24 °C. One day after recovery from hyperthermic stress (HS), they were given 60 ng/kg of bacterial endotoxin lipopolysaccharide (LPS) intravenously. Another group of rabbits were pretreated with oral antibiotics, and then submitted to the HS (Atbt+1-day post-HS/LPS) and LPS administration. Numbers of blood cells were counted.

Results and discussion
It was found (Figure 1) that the HS rabbits developed fever that was significantly higher than in normothermic rabbits (Control LPS). The Atbt+1-day post-HS/LPS rabbits did not exhibit any differences compared with the controls. Furthermore, rabbits pretreated with oral antibiotics without the HS (Control-Atbt/LPS) showed the same magnitude of LPS fevers as those of the control. Plasma LPS concentrations tended to be higher in the HS than in control animals. We also observed that white blood cell counts were higher in the HS than in control rabbits. It was reported that hyperthermic animals exhibit redistribution of blood from the core to the skin to facilitate heat loss (Hales et al., 1996). This can cause an ischemia in, e.g., the large intestine. Ensuing intestinal ischemia increases leakage of bacterial endotoxins into the blood through intestinal mucosal barrier (Hall et al., 2001). Present results may raise the question why animals become more susceptible to infections after they experienced HS (Sturm et al., 1989).

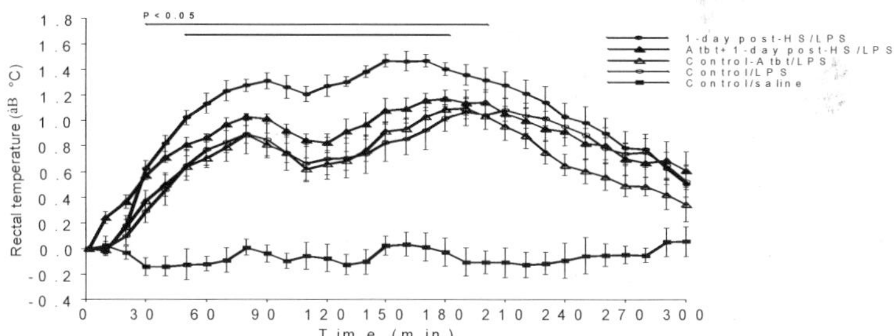

Figure 1. Rectal temperature changes in the experimental groups of rabbits with and without heat stress (HS) following intravenous LPS or 0.9% saline solution injections at time zero.

Conclusions
Enhanced LPS fevers in HS rabbits may be caused by leakage of a very small amount of LPS from the large intestine into blood circulation where it bounds with white blood cells. The increased number of white blood cells could become a diagnostic marker to assess the recovery of animals from the HS.

References
Hales J.R.S. et al., 1996. Handbook of Physiology, Section 4: Environmental Physiology. Oxford University Press, New York/Oxford. 285-355.

Hall D.M. et al., 2001. Am. J. Physiol. Heart Circ. Physiol. 280:509-521.

Sturm A.W. et al., 1989. Lancet 1: 968.

Heat stress parameters in Azawak (*Bos indicus*) and Modicana (*Bos taurus*) cattle

M. Zecchini[1*], S. Bordonaro[2], S. Barbieri[1], D. Marletta[2], G. D'Urso[2] & C. Crimella[1]
[1]*Istituto di Zootecnica, Facoltà di Medicina Veterinaria, Via G. Celoria, 10, 20133 Milano,* [2]*Dip. di Scienze Agronomiche, Agrochimiche e delle Produzioni Animali, via Valdisavoia, 5, 95123 Catania, Italy. massimo.zecchini@unimi.it*

Introduction

Hot environment heavily influences productive and reproductive traits of dairy cows. Objective measurements to describe heat stress adaptability are limited, but some metabolic and hematological parameters have been recommended (Gutierrez *et al.*, 1971; Hammond *et al.*, 1996 and 1998). The aim of this trial was to evaluate the effect of Temperature Humidity Index (THI) on heat stress parameters in Azawak (*Bos indicus*) and Modicana (*Bos taurus*) cattle, reared in each own environment.

Materials and methods

36 Azawak zebu cows in Niger and 30 Modicana cows in Sicilia reared under similar condition, were studied during 4 different periods. Rectal temperature (RT: °C) was recorded once a day (at max THI) for 7 days in each period. Blood samples were collected once a period to evaluate hemoglobin concentration (Hb: g/100 ml), Packed Cell Volume (PCV: %vol.) erythrocyte (EN: $10^6/mm^3$) and leukocyte (LN: $10^3/mm^3$) number, Mean Corpuscular Volume (MCV: μm^3) and Mean Corpuscular Hemoglobin (MCH: pg). Climatic measurements were recorded to calculate THI (Johnson, 1987). Data were analysed by the GLM procedure (SAS, 2000) with analysis of covariance.

Results and discussion

PCV, Hb, LN and MCH showed an high significant influence of individual variability ($P \leq 0.001$ for PCV, Hb, LN and $P \leq 0.01$ for MCH) and breed ($P \leq 0.001$ for PCV, Hb, LN and MCH). Effect of animal on EN, MCV and RT was not significant, while THI showed a significant influence (Table 1: $P \leq 0.001$ for EN, MCV and RT). The significant effect of breed could be affected by THI level; further investigations could point out the behavior of breed at the same THI.

Table 1. EN, MCV and RT (least square means ± standard error) in 4 periods.

	Azawak					Modicana				
	THI[a]	EN	MCV	THI[b]	RT	THI[a]	EN	MCV	THI[b]	RT
Period1	72.9	5.9±0.3	54.8±3.0	79.3	38.2±0.1	54.0	5.8±0.1	49.7±0.4	60.0	38.2±0.1
Period2	78.0	5.4±0.2	55.6±2.8	81.8	38.4±0.1	54.3	5.9±0.1	47.3±0.4	60.3	38.0±0.1
Period3	78.3	5.9±0.3	49.2±3.6	82.5	38.5±0.1	60.9	6.0±0.1	49.4±0.4	66.4	37.9±0.1
Period4	87.3	4.7±0.2	66.2±2.8	92.9	38.7±0.1	72.5	5.5±0.1	47.7±0.4	79.1	38.0±0.1

[a] mean values for each experimental period; [b] the mean of the highest values of each experimental period

Conclusions

Because of marginal influence of individual variability, EN, MCV and RT could be used in the assessment of hematological response to heat stress and they could be considered sharp indexes of heat stress tolerance. Our results pointed out EN, MCV and RT could be used to measure the response to heat stress condition and they might be introduced into selection program in hot climate.

References

Gutierrez J.H. *et al.*, 1971. J. Anim. Sci., 32:968-73.
Hammond A.C. *et al.*, 1996. J. Anim. Sci., 74:295-303.
Hammond *et al.*, 1998. J. Anim. Sci., 76:1568-77.
Johnson H.D., 1987. In: Bioclimatology and the adaptation of livestock. Elsevier, Amsterdam, NL.
SAS User's Guide. 2000. Version 8. SAS Institute, Inc., Cary, NC.

Acknowledgements

Research financed by Cofinanziamento MURST 1999.

Cooling non-lactating dairy cows reduces stress and improves postpartum performance

L. Avendaño-Reyes[1*], F.D. Alvarez-Valenzuela[1], A. Correa-Calderón[1], J.S. Saucedo-Quintero[1], F. Rivera-Acuña[1], F.J. Verdugo-Zárate[1], C.F. Aréchiga-Flores[2] & P.H. Robinson[3]
[1]Instituto de Ciencias Agrícolas, Universidad Autónoma de Baja California, Ej. Nuevo León, B.C., México, [2]Facultad de Medicina Veterinaria y Zootecnia, Universidad Autónoma de Zacatecas, Zac., México, [3]UCCE, Department of Animal Sciences, University of California, Davis, CA, USA. lar62@uabc.mx

Indroduction

High environmental heat decreases welfare of dairy cows and, in extreme situations, can lead to death.

Materials and methods

Physiological responses during the non-lactating (dry) period, as well as postpartum productive performance, to a cooling system were evaluated with 24 multiparous dry Holstein cows assigned to one of two groups at the beginning of their dry period being: with water spray and fans or with no cooling system. During the dry period, rectal temperature and respiration rate were taken twice a day (9:30 and 14:30 h) twice a week, body condition score was recorded once a week and a blood sample was collected to be analyzed for thyroid hormones. Post-partum variables collected were calf birth weight, milk production and composition, and reproduction parameters. Data were analyzed using a repeated mesures design and Chi-square analysis.

Results and discussion

Average daytime high and low temperatures during the period of study were 48°C and 23°C. Cooled cows had a lower ($P<0.05$) respiration rate (77.5 vs. 84.4 breaths/min) and rectal temperature (39.1 vs. 39.3 °C) at 14:30 h, and higher body condition (BC) score ($P<0.05$) overall (4.03 vs. 3.92 BC units). Plasma thyroxine and triiodothyronine levels were higher ($P<0.05$) in cooled cows (37.1 vs. 30.0 ng/ml and 0.81 vs. 0.69 ng/ml) indicating reduced stress. Calf birth weights showed a trend ($P=0.15$) to be higher in cooled cows (35.7 vs. 32.9 kg). Milk yield at week eight of lactation was higher ($P<0.05$) for the cooled group (28.2 vs. 26.4 kg/d). However, milk fat and protein proportions were similar, as well as total milk yield. Conception rate was higher ($P<0.05$) in cooled cows (100 vs. 64%) and culling rate was lower through the end of the lactation (0 vs. 48.3%). Economic analysis showed that net benefits of cooling represented a benefit of US$75/cow. Results show that cooling dry cows using fans with water spray reduced cow stress, and improved welfare, under these very hot conditions. However, post-partum productive performance was generally not affected, although reproductive performance was enhanced.

Conclusions

Overall benefits resulted in a substantial net positive economic benefit.

References

Collier R.J. et al., 1982. J. Anim. Sci. 54:309-319.
Lewis G.S. et al., 1984. J. Anim. Sci. 58:174-186.
Moore R.B. et al., 1992. J. Dairy Sci. 75:1877-1883.
SAS Institute Inc., 1986. SAS for linear models. A guide to the ANOVA and GLM procedures. Pp 82-83. Cary, NC.
Wolfenson D. et al., 1988. J. Dairy Sci. 71:809-818.

Use of different shelter in summer for dairy sheep: lamb birth and weaning weight

L. Biondi[1*], G. Cascone[2], G. Piccione[3] & P. Pennisi[1]
[1]*D.A.C.P.A., Università di Catania,* [2]*D.I.A., Università di Catania,* [3]*Dipartimento Mo. Bi. Fi. Pa., Università di Messina, Italy. lubiondi@mbox.fagr.unict.it*

Introduction

Typical sheep breeding system in Sicily requires ewes to conclude pregnancy and start lactation in summer. Literature reveals the negative effects of heat stress on reproductive performance of ruminants: reduced placental growth in ewes (McCrabb and Bortolussi, 1996) and lamb birth weight (McCrabb et al., 1993); reduced content in immunoglobulins in cows colostrum (Lacetera, 1998).

Materials and methods

Two groups of 14 pluriparous pregnant (~4th month) Comisana ewes were housed in two different shelters from July to September. Indoor Group (IG) were allowed to use an open sheep-fold with an outside paddock; Outdoor Group (OG) a fenced area shaded with a net. At lambing (throughout August) and at weaning (30 d post lambing), ewe live weight (LW) and body condition score (BCS, 0-5 scale), and lamb live weight were recorded. 50 ml of individual colostrum were collected for γ–globulins determination. Air temperature, speed and relative humidity in each housing type were recorded; THI was calculated. Lamb data were analyzed by a model including 3 effects: type of shelter, type of parturition and sex. Colostrum data were analysed by a model including just the effect of shelter, as well as ewe live weight and BCS data.

Results and discussion

Average hourly THI index was similar in the two conditions: minimum THI was about 67 and was performed at 06.00 a.m.; maximum THI was about 78 and was performed at 02.00 p.m. Outdoor shelter was much more ventilated: greater differences in air speed were recorded between 12.00 a.m and 08.00 p.m., ranging from 2 to 5 ms^{-1}. Ewe LW and BCS at lambing and at weaning were not affected by the experimental factor (table 1). γ–globulins percentage was not affected by the experimental factor, too. Lamb LW was, obviously, affected either by type of lambing and sex. Lamb LW was significantly affected by type of shelter used by their mothers during the last weeks of pregnancy and the first weeks of lactation. Both birth and 30 d LW were higher in outdoor lambs ($P< 0.05$).

Table 1. Principal results.

	Ewes weight, kg		Ewes BCS		Colostrum	Lambs weight, kg	
	lambing	30 d	lambing	30 d	γ-glob., %	birth	30 d
Indoor	57.6	55.3	2.95	2.79	50.69	3.81 a	10.95 a
Outdoor	56.1	55.0	2.92	2.90	48.70	4.19 b	11.55 b

a, b = P<0.05

Conclusions

The ventilation created a microclimatic condition that, probably, gave higher welfare in OG ewes compared with IG ones. Shading net appears to be an interesting and cheap shelter during summer season in Mediterranean areas.

References

McCrabb G.J. and Bortolussi G., 1996. Small Ruminant Res. 20:121-127.
McCrabb G.J. et al., 1993. Austr. J. Agric. Res. 44:933-943.
Lacetera N., 1998. Zoot. Nutr. Anim. 24:239-246.

Shade effects on physiological responses of feeder cattle

T.M. Brown-Brandl*, R.A. Eigenberg, J.A. Nienaber & G.L. Hahn
USDA-ARS-MARC, Clay Center, NE 68933, USA. brandl@email.marc.usda.gov

Introduction

Heat stress in cattle causes decreases in feed intake and growth, and in extreme cases can cause death. An extreme event in July, 1995, caused the loss of approximately 3,750 head of cattle in western Iowa; direct losses were estimated at $2.8 million and production losses at $28 million (Busby et al., 1996). Shade has been shown to reduce direct and indirect losses in some areas of the country. Shades have consistently provided a reduction in core body temperature and respiration rate of cattle (Mitloehner et al., 1999; Valtorta et al., 1997). During times of high solar radiation, temperature, and high humidity, a reduction of solar radiation may be a method of reducing heat stress (Blackshaw et al., 1994). The objective of this report was to further evaluate the physiological responses of feedlot cattle to shade during summer conditions.

Materials and methods

Eight crossbred steers (initially weighing 294.7±10.8 kg) were randomly assigned to one of eight individual pens where one of two treatments was applied; shade (S), or no shade (NS). Data were collected during seven, 5-day periods. The steers changed treatments each period. Respiration rate (RR), feed intake (FI), and core body temperature (t_{core}) were collected using automated systems. Shade preference data were evaluated using video recordings. Weather data were collected from an automated weather data center located within 1.5 km of the pens. The data were categorized by daily maximum temperature (Hot days t_{max} >34.5°C [7 days]; Cool days t_{max} <28.4°C [5 days]). Hourly data for hot and cool days were analyzed using the general linear model procedure in SAS (SAS, 2000) for effects of animal (A), treatment (TRT), period (P), hr, and the interaction of TRT and hr (TRT*hr).

Results and discussion

Although not statistically compared, the pattern of physiological responses on hot and cool days differed greatly. On cool days, RR and t_{core} were significantly affected by A, P, hr, TRT*hr, where on hot days TRT had a significant influence also. Upon closer investigation, S had only a slight advantage on cool days; during daytime hours (1000 – 1900 hr), S cattle had RR 3.3 bpm lower, t_{core} 0.09°C lower, and 0.50 kg more FI than the NS cattle. However, on hot days S had a large impact; between the hours of 1000 – 1900 hr, S cattle had RR 25.4 bpm lower, t_{core} 0.5°C lower, and 1.86 kg more FI. The use of shade between cool and hot days didn't differ significantly (cool days – 81% vs. hot days – 95%).

Conclusions

Shade was beneficial on cool and hot days; as expected, the beneficial effects were much greater on hot days. Between the hours of 1000 - 1900 on the hot days, shade reduced RR by over 25 bpm and t_{core} by 0.5 °C. Feed intake was 1.86 kg greater in the shade.

References

Blackshaw J.K. et al., 1994. Aust. J. Exp. Agric. 34:285-295. Busby F. et al., 1996. Heat Stress in Feedlot Cattle: Producer Survey Results. Beef Research Report , A.S. Leaflet R1348. Iowa State University, Ames, IA.

Mitloehner et al., 1999. J. Anim. Sci. 77:148. SAS User's Guide. 2000. Version 8. SAS Institute, Inc., Cary, NC. Valtorta S. et al., 1997. Int'l. J. Biomet. 41:65-67.

Productive and metabolic response of dairy cows raised in barn equipped with fans and misters during the summer season

L. Calamari[1*], M. Speroni[2], E. Frazzi[3], L. Stefanini[4] & G. Licitra[5]
[1]Istituto di Zootecnica, Facoltà di Agraria, 29100 Piacenza, [2]Istituto Sperimentale per la Zootecnia, 26100 Cremona, [3]Istituto di Genio Rurale, Facoltà di Agraria, 29100 Piacenza, [4]Azienda Sperimentale "V. Tadini, 29027 Podenzano, Piacenza, [5]Corfilac, 97100 Ragusa, Italy. luigi.calamari@unicatt.it

Introduction

A reduction of heat stress in dairy cattle sheds has been obtained using ventilation with misting or sprinkling. Our aim was to evaluate the effect of ventilation and misting on physiological and productive response of dairy cows in southern Italy.

Materials and methods

The trial was carried out during two consecutive years (May to September) in four barns. In each barn the lactating cows were housed in two pens designated as control (C) with no cooling and treated (T) equipped with fans along the feed alley (switched on at 25°C). Two misters (0.3 l/min) were in front of each fan and activated at 26.5°C (60'' of misting every 180'', increased by 6'' for each 1°C over 26.5°C). Microclimatic parameters were monitored continuously and DMI was recorded daily. On 10 cows per group weekly controls were performed on milk yield (MY), breathing rate (BR) and rectal temperature (RT), and monthly for blood parameters (Bertoni et al., 1998).

Results and discussion

BR and RT were lower in T group, in relation to the better microclimatic conditions (lower air temperature and higher wind speed), whereas THI was similar in the 2 pens. The higher heat stress in C affected negatively DMI ($P<0.001$) in the 1st year (-1.1 and -2.23 kg/head/d in farm 1 and 2 respectively) and MY. Lower values of plasma cholesterol and alkaline phosphatase (ALP) in C seems to confirm the higher heat stress in C group (Calamari et al., 1997; Ronchi et al., 1997). The variability of the urea levels was mainly related to the different protein content of the diets (from 15.5 to 18.4% on DM) and the lower urea values observed in C seems partially related to the lower DMI.

Table 1. BR, RT, DMI, MY and plasma parameters (cholesterol, ALP and urea) in C and T.

Farm (year)	1 (1999)		2 (1999)		3 (2000)		4 (2000)	
	C	T	C	T	C	T	C	T
THI_{max}	78.87	78.34	80.10	80.50	76.62	77.43	77.10	77.70
BR (n/min)	67.05^B	59.79^A	79.54^b	70.70^a	71.42	69.78	67.42^b	59.54^a
RT (T°)	39.23^B	38.77^A	38.99	38.88	38.75	38.83	38.72	38.67
MY (kg/d)	31.89	33.30	30.50^A	33.56^B	27.00	29.21	38.90	41.45
Chol. (mmol/l)	6.07	6.50	5.69	6.35	6.32^a	7.09^b	6.45	6.78
ALP (U/l)	31.62^a	39.54^b	40.27	39.24	39.73	43.68	37.62^a	48.06^b
Urea (mmol/l)	6.86	7.02	5.99	5.76	6.07	6.34	6.42^a	7.25^b

a,b: $P<0.05$; A, B: $P<0.001$

Conclusions

From our results we can conclude that an environmental conditioning system can improve the animal response to hot conditions in southern Italy. The variations of cholesterol and ALP could be used to evaluate the animal response to the hot conditions.

References

Bertoni et al., 1998, Zoot. Nutr. Anim., 24: 17-29.
Calamari L. et al., 1996. Atti SISVet, 50: 491-492.
Ronchi B. et al., 1997, Zoot. Nutr. Anim., 23: 3-15.

Acknowledgements

Research supported by POM. Misura 2, A/9.

The effect of a combined progesterone (PRID) and ovosynch protocol on pregnancy rate in Buffalo

F. De Rensis*[1], G. Ronci[1], P. Guarneri[1], A. Patelli[1], G.M. Bettoni[1] & B.X. Nguyen[2]
[1]Dipartimento di Salute Animale, Facoltà di Medicina Veterinaria, Parma, Italy, [2]Lab. of Biol. of Reprod. and Develop., National Center for Sciences and Technology, Hanoi, Vietnam. fabio.derensis@unipr.it

Introduction

It is possible to synchronize ovulation in buffaloes for artificial insemination during breeding season, however, the efficacy of treatments can be compromised by the season. In dairy cattle it has been demonstrated that the success of a ovosinc+TAI program is dependent on whether the cows are cycling as well as the stage of the oestrous cycle at the time of ovosync /TAI protocol. In seasonally anoestrous suckled beef cows treatment with progesterone can initiate cyclicity. Therefore this study was designed to evaluate in buffalo the effect of progesterone administration to a timed insemination protocols during the low breeding season.

Materials and methods

Between April and August 2002, 28 buffaloes (GPG group) were treated with GnRH (d0) (Cystoreline® 100µg/cow, im, CEVA Vetem, Italy), seven days later (d7) with $PGF_{2\alpha}$ (alfaprostol 8 mg/cow, im, Gabrostim®, CEVAVetem) followed 48h later with GnRH (d9). Fixed time insemination was made 12 to 16 hours after the end of the protocol. Another 37 buffaloes (GPG+PRID group) were treated as in group GPG with the adjunct of Progesterone Releasing Intravaginal Device for 7 days (PRID®, CEVA Vetem Italy, without oestradiol capsule) beginning the day of the first GnRH administration. Ovarian activity was evaluated by rectal and ultrasound examination.

Results and discussion

The overall pregnancy rate in GPG group was 35.7% (10/28), in GPG+PRID group 44.7% (17/38) (Table 1). When it is considered the effect of treatment in animals with no ovarian activity, the pregnancy rate in the GPG group was 1/7 (14.2%) and in GPG+PRID group was 4/10 (40.0%) (Tab 1)

Table 1. Pregnancy rate after ovosinc/TAI protocol with (GPG+PRID) or without (GPG) progesterone administration for 7 days in buffaloes during the low breeding season.

Treatments	n°	mean BCS	n°of calving	Pregnancy rate
Group GPG				
cycling	21	3.2±0.4	3.8±1.9	9/21(42.8%)
not cycling	7	3.4±0.6	4.0±1.2	1/7 (14.2%)
total	28	3.12±0.1	3.8±2.1	10/28(35.7%)
Group GPG+PRID				
cycling	28	3.1±0.2	3.2±1.1	13/28(46.4%)
not cycling	10	3.1±0.4	3.4±1.9	4/10(40.0%)
total	38	3.1±0.43	3.3±1.7	17/38 (44.7%)

Conclusions

The results shown that in anestrous buffaloes during low breeding season pregnancy rate after treatment with GnRH/PGF/GnRH and timed artificial insemination can be improved by the use of a progestrone intravaginal device.

Acknowledgements

This research was supported by Ministero degli Esteri, Italia, (legge 401/1990, prog. S&T Italia-Vietnam 2002-205, prot n°269/1966) and FIL 2001. We thank CEVA VETEM, Italy, for providing Cystoreline®, PRID and Gabrostim.

Cooling of dairy cows in Israel - Improving cows welfare and performance as well as reducing environmental contamination

I. Flamenbaum[1*], E. Shoshani[1] & E. Ezra[2]

[1]Ministry of agriculture, Extension service, POB 28 Beit-Dagan,, Israel, 50250, [2]Israel Cattle Breeders Association, Caesariya, Israel. israflam@shaham.moag.gov.il

Introduction

Production and fertility of Israeli cows are negatively affected by summer conditions. Summer milk production reaches only 85% of winter level. Conception Rates of cows inseminated in summer and winter are 20% and 50% respectively. Cooling cows in Israel is based mainly on wetting and forced ventilation and creates serious environmental problems. The presented work studied: 1) the effect of intensive cooling in summer on cows welfare and performance and 2) the effect of different wetting methods and amount of water used on cooling efficiency and environmental contamination.

Materials and methods

Study 1: The effect of cooling dairy cows was studied by a large scale survey realized during four years (1998–2001), included 11 farms located in the costal part of Israel, classified into two groups according to the use of cooling in summer. Cows in group 1 (intensive cooling, six farms) were cooled in the holding and feeding area for a total of 10 cooling periods and 7.5 cumulative hours per day. Each cooling period combined cycles of sprinkling (0.5 min, 100 lit/h sprinklers) and forced ventilation (4.5 min.). Cows in group 2 (no cooling, five farms) were not cooled at all and served as a control group.

Study 2: Compared the effect of intensive cooling of cows in summer using a combination of forced ventilation and wetting the cows by two wetting methods. Cows in "method 1" were wetted as described in study 1. Cows in "method 2" were wetted by low-pressure misters (7 l/h mister). Four misters were located in front of each fan installed in the feeding area. Both groups received 10 cooling periods and 7.5 cumulative hours daily as in study 1. Amount of water used for cooling in "method 2" group was les than half of that used in "method 1", help to maintain feeding area surface of this group drier.

Results

Study 1: Milk production (kg/d) and conception rates (%) were calculated for summer (July-September) and winter (December-February). The analysis included 125,000 milk recordings and 17,000 first inseminations. Average four years daily low and high temperatures (°C) were 8.4 and 19.3, and 22.0 and 31.8, for winter and summer, respectively. The interaction between season and cooling system was significant ($P<0.001$). The ratios between summer and winter production were 98.5% and 93.4%, in intensive cooled and no cooled primiparous cows and 98.5%, and 90.7% in multiparous cows, respectively. Conception-rates were 55.8%, 53.9%, 40.4%, and 14.6%, for primiparous cows under the intensive cooling and no cooling regimes, inseminated in winter and summer, respectively ($P<0.01$). Conception-rates were 46.6%, 43.5%, 33.8% and 16.7% for multiparous cows in the same groups inseminated in winter and summer, respectively ($P<0.01$).

Study 2: Average daily Temperature-Humidity Index (THI) ranged during the summer between 70 and 76 and was above critical level most of the day. Cows in both groups were normothermic during most of the day (38.8 °c and 38.6 °c for cows in methods 1 and 2 respectively). Production and conception–rate did not differ between treatments. Average milk production per cow during the experimental period (July–October) was 40.1 and 40.5 kg/d for cows wetted in methods 1 and 2 respectively. Conception–rate in first inseminations of the same groups and the same period were 54% and 59% respectively.

Conclusions

Intensive cooling of cows in summer, based on wetting and force ventilation reduced great part of summer decline in milk production and fertility. Replacing sprinklers by low-pressure misters in feeding area, reduced amount of water used and feeding area surface wetting level without affecting cows welfare and performance.

Behaviour of dairy cows in hot season in a barn equipped with automatic milking system (AMS)

E. Frazzi* & F. Calegari
Istituto di Genio Rurale, Università Cattolica del Sacro Cuore, Via Emilia Parmense, 84 – 29100 PC, Italy. ist.geniorurale-pc@unicatt.it

Introduction

It was considered that the hot conditions create different problems on the cows productivity and physiology (Bernabucci et al., 1998; Bertoni, 1998; Frazzi et al., 2002), in addition it disturbs their activities. We have set up an AMS (Automatic Milking System) in a barn to verify the influence of heat stress on the behaviour of the cows.
The study of the behaviour of the cows during the hot period could allow the improvement of the inside distribution of the barn and especially, it could give a useful indication on the planning and dislocation of the climatization system.

Materials and methods

The research has been carried out in an Italian breeding site, from mid July to mid August of 2002, equipped with AMS and conditioned with fans and misters. The herd of 49 lactating cows with a robotic station, has been monitored with digital videocamera, moreover, microclimatic parameter has been collected. It has been evaluated the presence of the cows in the varied sectors of the barn (milking, feeding and resting) continuously during the day with videocamera recording a 1 second every minute.

Results and discussion

The summer season during which the study has been carried out was not particularly hot. The maximum temperature during the whole study period with in the barn has been recorded 30°C only in three occasions. In the milking parlour the maximum presence of the cows was observed in the hours near feeds delivery and the values decreased as air temperature increased (Table 1). In the hotter days the cows tend to stay for a longer period in the feeding area reducing the number of the passages across the robotic station. This creates a problem from the self-milking point of view and the intervention of the operators is necessary.

Table 1. Cows (%) in the milking parlour in relation to the minimum daily temperature.

T. Min (°C)	Hour			
	24.00 – 06.00	06.00 – 12.00	12.00 – 18.00	18.00 – 24.00
< 21.5	2.36	5.07	2.79	4.93
	(*)	**		(*)
>21.5	1.36	3.58	2.34	3.77

(*) = P<0.1; **= P<0.01.

Conclusions

The results demonstrated, as it was expected, a reduction of the presences of cows in the milking parlour in the days with more elevated temperatures. The defence from the heat stress is important in all the barn, particularly in a barn equipped with AMS, where the activity of the animals is fundamental to the aim of the self-milking. In the robotic barns and in the areas with hot climate, as those in Italy, the realization of an effective conditioning system is fundamental for a better operation within the barn.

References

Bernabucci U. et al., 1998. Zoot. Nutr. Anim. 24:247-258.
Bertoni G., 1998. Zoot. Nutr. Anim. 24:273-282.
Frazzi E. et al., 2002. Transaction ASAE 45(2):395-405.

Effect of short-term cooling on some physiological responses of buffaloes. 1. Pregnant buffaloes

H.H. Khalifa[1*], M.M. Youssef[2] & M.M. Ghoneim[2]
[1]Department of Animal Production, Faculty of Agriculture, Al-Azhar University, Nasr City, Cairo, Egypt, [2]Animal Production Research Institute, Dokki, Giza, Egypt. khalifahhk@usa.net

Introduction

The majority of buffalo animals habitat tropical and sub-tropical climates of the world. In Egypt, there are about 3.1 million head of buffalo animals which comprises the most important source of livestock production in the country. There are lack of information regarding the impacts of heat stress on milk productivity, reproductive efficiency and metabolic rate of buffaloes. The present work aims to study the physiological respones of short-term cooling on alleviation of the environmental heat stress on pregnant buffaloes and the expected responses on their performance.

Materials and methods

Twelve buffalos were chosen at late pregnancy period to study the impacts of heat stress and short-term cooling during the period from June to September. The animals raised in a state farm located in the north of Nile delta where, the maximum ambient temperature ranged between 34.30 °C to 37.11 °C and the difference between THI values during day and night was 17.93 on average. The average LBW of cooled (DT) and non cooled (DC) pregnant buffaloes were 550 and 523 kg, respectively. The treated group was subjected to water-cooling system using an array of 16 static sprinklers dispatched within four water lines in paved restricted area. Skin temperature (ST), rectal temperature (RT) and respiration rate (RR) of each of the experimental animals were measured just before time of sprinkling (at 12 p.m.) and once again after cooling program (at 4 p.m.).

Results and discussion

The effects of cooling and month of testing on all parameters of adaptive response were highly significant ($P<0.01$). Comparing the estimates of adaptive responses taken at 12.00 a.m. with those taken at 4.00 p.m., ST, RT and RR of group DT decreased by 0.66 °C, 0.67 °C and 2.27 Respir./ min. On the other side, ST, RT and RR of group DC increased by 0.87 °C, 0.73 C° and 2.86 Respir./ min, respectively.

Month of sampling had a significant effect ($P<0.01$) on blood Hb and PCV% of buffaloes with no obvious difference between the cooled or non-cooled groups. Month of sampling had no effect on any of the tested blood metabolites. Blood total proteins or its fractions, blood urea nitrogen (BUN), total lipids and thyroid hormones (T3 and T4) were significantly higher ($P<0.05$) in the cooled animals. Higher estimates of gain/TDN intake were attained by the cooled group DT than DC group. The average daily milk yield of group DT was greater by 10.68 % than that of DC group. The number of days open were not distinctly different whereas, the number of services per conception were optimally 1.37 for group DT versus 1.75 for group DC.

Conclusions

Short-term cooling anticipated in reducing the summer heat load of pregnant buffaloes till time of delivery such that they were subjected for the subsequent mating in the moderate climate of autumn.

References

Her E. et al., 1988. J. Dairy Sci. 71(4):1085-1092.

Flamenbaum I. et al., 1995. J. Dairy Sci. 78(10): 2221-2229.

The covers for animals' protection in warm areas

A. Gusman[1*], A. Marucci[1] & C. Bibbiani[2]
[1]Dipartimento D.A.F. Università degli Studi dellaTuscia, 01100 Viterbo, [2]Dipartimento dell'Ambiente Agroforestale, Università degli Studi di Pisa, Italy. gusman@unitus.it

Introduction

The main problem in the southern regions of the Mediterranean countries during the summer season, is the high intensity of solar radiation which, combined with the contemporary high air temperature, makes it difficult to put into effect safe and efficient systems of protections able to make the environment suitable for the breeding of animals like the dairy cows.
To oppose this phenomenon the materials of the covers of the structures of breeding must have certain physical features as the weight, reflectivity, and thermo conductivity suitable to contrast and delay the flow of energy generated by the solar radiation.
The research carried out with different typologies of covers for verifying the efficiency and for drawing out a model of mathematical simulation of the phenomenon.

Materials and methods

Different typologies of covers have been tested. They have been of single layer, of two layers and of more layers composed by current materials as tiles, steel asbestos cement, wood. Prototypes of the size of about 4m have been created.
Thermometric probes connected to a Data logger have monitored them.

Results and discussion

The lowest value of the internal face, under the single layer roofing shelters never goes below about 53°C while with the simple adding of an expanded polyurethane layer, the temperature of the internal face goes down to values which are little higher than 40°-41°C.
Really, better results are obtained with roofing shelters formed by zinc-plated steel polished plates + polyurethane + wood + clay tiles + air space + wood.
In both cases under the roofing shelters the temperature of the internal parameter is lower, even of very little, than the highest temperature of the air (-0,4°C e 0,6°C).
Moreover the phase-difference reaches about 2 h and if it cannot be considered entirely as the optimum it is surely meaningful and it is the best that can be obtained with these simple materials.

Conclusions

The use of simple layer (only sheet- steel or tiles or asbestos cement plates) covers must be surely excluded in the regions with a Mediterranean climate with a high solar radiation for a long period of the year.
A considerable improvement can be obtained by adding a layer of insulating material like the expanded polyurethane to these covers and by using colours close to white.
The best performances ,as we expected, have been with the triple layer covers and especially for those in which the use of a wood plateau has been provided.

References

Pitts D.R. & Sissom L.E., 1977. Heat Transfer, McGraw-Hill Book Company, New York. Jui Sheng Hsieh P.E., 1986. Solar Energy Engineering. Prentice-hall, Inc, Englewood Cluiffs, New Jersey.
Duffie J.A. & Beckman W.A., 1991. Solar engineering of thermal process. John Wiley & Sons, Inc. New York. AA.VV. 1986. Nuovo Colombo - Manuale dell'Ingegnere. Ed. Hoepli, Milano.

Behavior of crossbred lactating cows grazing *Pennisetum purpureum*, Schumaker in Southeastern Brazil under two feeding systems

L. P. Novaes[1]*, M. F. A. Pires[1], C. L. Werneck[2] & R. S. Verneque[1]
[1]*Embrapa Dairy Cattle Research Center – Rua Eugênio do Nascimento, 610 Dom Bosco, Juiz de Fora, MG Brazil,* [2]*Universidade Federal de Juiz de Fora, MG Brazil. novaes@cnpgl.embrapa.br*

Introduction

Ingestive behavior of cattle is affected by several factors and hot or cold weather, can increase maintenance requirements (Grant et al., 2001). This study measured elephantgrass grazing time (GT), ruminating (RUM) and idling (REST) times when standing or lying down of crossbred cows under two management systems.

Material and methods

The experiment was carried out at the National Dairy Cattle Research Center in Cel. Pacheco, MG-Brazil (21° 33' 22'' south latitude, 43° 06' 15'' west longitude, 430 m altitude). Climate is classified as Cwa (KÖPPEN). Four paddocks (720 m^2 each), with fertilized elephantgrass (N=200, K_2O/ha/year), were rotationally grazed, three/thirty days grazing resting periods, stocked at 5 AU (AU=450 kg LW). Cows' behavior was measured by immediate observation (Martin et al., 1986), two observation/cow (eight observations/season). Eight cows were randomly split into four groups and then submitted to treatments: T1= elephantgrass pasture (EP) and T2= EP + 1.0 kg/day/cow of concentrate fed to each 2.0 kg of milk produced above 10 kg, milked at 07:00 and 14:00h. All cows were corn silage supplemented (30 kg/day/cow) in winter.. Analyses of variance included period (day= 6:00-18:00h/night= 18:00- 6:00h), season (summer/winter), treatments (with/without concentrate) and their interactions as fixed effects.

Results and discussion

GT was significant ($P<0.05$) for day period with 5h 15min (day) x 3h 12min (night), and the day period*season and grazing period*season interactions. Day period and day period*season interaction affected GT with cows showing a diurnal grazing pattern. From 8h 27min, 61% of this time was day grazing, result is in accordance with those from Fraser et al., (1990) and Lima et al., (1999). Average RUM time was 3h 09min, being affected by day period*season. Standing was the position by cows spent more time RUM during winter and lying down in summer. Independent of position cows spent more time RUM at night ($P<0.05$). Total REST time was 9h 57min which is in the range cited in literature (Costa, 2000). Time spent in REST (standing or lying down) was affected by day period*season interaction ($P<0.05$). Day REST in standing position was higher ($P<0.05$) in winter than summer (2h 26min x 54min), being different of data from Shultz, (1983), however, cows were in a paved floor between milking and probably this could have induced them to stand instead of lying down.

Conclusions

In hot days cows tended to alter their ingestive behavior, with minimum grazing from 11h until 15 h.

References

Costa M. J. R., 2000. Pelotas: UFP, 168 p. MSc Thesis.
Fraser A.F. et al., 1990. Farm animal behavior and welfare. 3ed, London: Balliere Tindall, 437 p.
Grant R. J. et al., 2001 . J. Dairy Sci. 84(E. Suppl.):E156-163.
Lima M.L.P. et al., 1999. In: Reunião Anual da Sociedade Brasileira de Zootecnia, 31 Porto Alegre. Anais. Porto Alegre RS: Sociedade Brasileira de Zootecnia.
Martin P. et al., 1986. Measuring behavior: an introdutore guide. Cambridge: University Press, 200 p.
Shultz T. A., 1983. J. Dairy Sci. 67:868-873.

Effects of silymarin on rumen metabolism and microbial population in goats exposed to hot environment

G. Acuti[1*], S. Costarelli[2], I. Tomassetti[1], E. Chiaradia[1], L. Avellini[1] & M. Trabalza-Marinucci[1]
[1]Dipartimento di Tecnologie e Biotecnologie delle Produzioni Animali, Università degli Studi di Perugia, 06126 Perugia, Italy, [2]Istituto Zooprofilattico Sperimentale dell'Umbria e delle Marche, Perugia, Italy. vete3@unipg.it

Introduction

Ruminants react to heat stress by decreasing DM intake and gastro-intestinal passage rate. Silymarin extract is reported to protect liver cells and to provide antioxidant, immune stimulating and anti-inflammatory effects (Wellington et al., 2001), which can be of value during heat stress. No information is available on the effect of silymarin on rumen metabolism. The aim of this paper was to investigate the effects of silymarin on goats exposed to hot environment in climatic chambers.

Materials and methods

Nine non-pregnant non-lactating Saanen goats were allocated by randomised block design to receive one of three dietary treatments. The control (C) group was fed an *ad lib* diet based hay wafers (78%) and mixed concentrate. The other 2 groups received either 400 (S1) or 800 mg silymarin/d (S2). Animals were kept under thermal comfort (THI = 62) for the first 14 d (P1), then exposed to heat stress (THI = 76-84) for 21 d (P2) and finally returned to thermal comfort for 21 d (P3). At the end of each period a sample of rumen contents was taken via stomach tube and analysed for pH, protozoa and bacteria number, NH_3, lactate and VFA. Data were subjected to ANOVA.

Results and discussion

Microbial population did not appear to be affected by heat stress, except for protozoa whose concentration increased throughout P2 and P3. NH_3 concentration was shown to be decreased by heat stress, as observed by Shafie et al. (1994) in sheep. Silymarin decreased cellulolytic bacterial numbers; this effect was confirmed by *in vitro* trials (data not shown). If silymarin has to be used to alleviate heat stress in ruminants, further studies are needed to elucidate its role in rumen metabolism.

Table 1. Rumen parameters as affected by heat stress and silymarin treatment.

	Treatment				THI			*THI*
	C	S1	S2	*SE*	P1	P2	P3	*SE*
Bacteria/ml (log)								
Total	8.22	8.05	7.89	*0.19*	8.18	8.17	7.83	*0.19*
Amylolitic	7.62	8.02	7.72	*0.20*	7.98	7.86	7.52	*0.20*
Cellulolitic	8.06 a	7.47 b	7.36 b	*0.30*	7.53	7.33	-	*0.22*
Protozoa ($x10^5$/ml)	6.04	5.45	6.21	*0.62*	4.46 A	5.72 B	7.54 C	*0.62*
VFA (mM)	75.41	70.04	67.75	*10.70*	65.64	68.29	79.28	*10.70*
NH_3 (mg/dl)	15.52	15.16	18.95	*1.20*	16.04 a	15.29 b	18.30 a	*1.20*
Lactate (mM)	0.37	0.40	0.34	*0.04*	0.34	0.39	0.38	*0.04*

a, b: P<0.05; A, B: P<0.01

References

Shafie M.M. et al., 1994. Egypt. J. Anim. Prod. 71:258-263.
Wellington K. et al., 2001. BioDrugs 15:465-89.

Acknowledgements

The Department of Animal Productions of the University of Viterbo is gratefully acknowledged for helpful assistance throughout the experiment.

CH_4 emissions from cubicle houses on dairy farms with advanced nutrient management

J.W.H. Huis in 't Veld & G.J. Monteny*
Institute for Agricultural and Environmental Engineering (IMAG), Report 2003-01, Wageningen, the Netherlands. gert-jan.monteny@wur.nl

Introduction
In the Netherlands, dairy farmers are forced to comply with losses of nutrients in the framework of the Mineral Account System (MINAS). In a national project, a selected numbers of farmers are encouraged to further improve their nutrient management, in order to reduce losses beyond the legislative levels. One of the questions raised was if this would also influence the emission of methane (CH_4) from the animal houses, since dietary measures are on of the options envisaged.

Materials and methods
A monitoring study was conducted on 9 of the participating farms. Methane emissions were measured with a combination of a trace gas system to calculate the ventilation rate, and auto-filling air containers, placed in the top of the building, to measure the CH_4 concentration accumulated with time. Measurement periods lasted approximately 4 weeks per farm.

Results and discussion
The results are shown in the figure below, where the measurements are compared with calculated CH_4 emissions based on normative emission factors relative to milk yield (14 g CH_4 per kg of milk and day) and dry matter intake (24 g CH_4 per kg of dry matter from roughage and 20 g from concentrates; Veen, 2001). Measured CH_4 emissions range 310-670 g/animal per day (average: 501). Milk yield (408-521 g; average 461g) and dry matter intake (474-699 g; average 590 g) appeared to respectively under estimate (8%) and over estimate (18%) the measured emissions

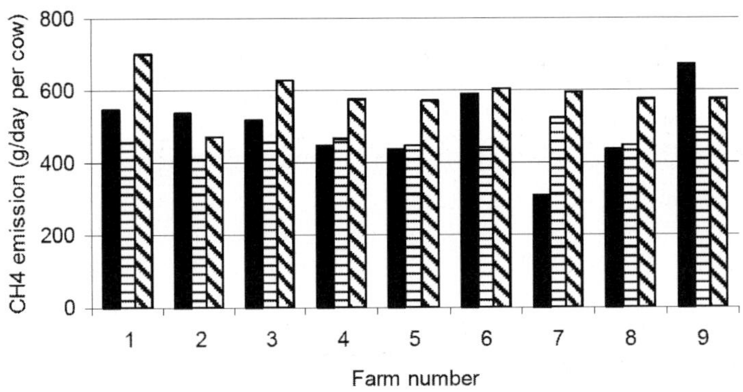

Conclusions
Measured CH_4 emissions from dairy cow houses appear to be greater than default values used in international emission inventories (e.g. IPCC). A combination of milk yield and dry matter intake can be a reliable predictor for the CH_4 emissions from dairy cow houses.

References
Huis in 't Veld J.W.H. and Monteny G.J., 2003. IMAG report 2003-01, Wageningen, the Netherlands, 42.
Veen W.A.G., 2001. Institute for Animal Nutrition 'De Schothorst', Lelystad, the Netherlands, 56.

Effects of elevated atmospheric carbon dioxide concentration on floristic composition and forage quality of a Mediterranean grassland

A. Raschi[1*], A. Martini[2], A. Pezzati[2], F. Albanito[2], M. Lanini[1] & F. Selvi[3]
[1]C.N.R.-IBIMET, 50145 Firenze, Italy, [2]Dip. di Scienze Zootecniche, Università di Firenze, 50144 Firenze, Italy, [3]Dip. Biologia Vegetale, Università di Firenze, 50144 Firenze, Italy. raschi@ibimet.cnr.it

Introduction

The ongoing global changes have been demonstrated to affect growth, phenology and chemical composition of plants (Raschi et al., 1997); as the response has been proved to be species-specific, changes are expected in the specific composition of plant communities (Leadley et al., 1996). This research aimed to investigate the response of a semi-natural Mediterranean grassland to the current increase in atmospheric carbon dioxide concentration, to test how it will affect the structure and botanical composition, the growth and productivity, and the forage quality.

Materials and methods

The experiment was performed in Rapolano Terme (Central Italy, Siena Province). In a semi-natural grassland a FACE (Free Air CO_2 Enrichment) setup was installed. It consisted of six carbon dioxide fumigation rings (FR), plus six identical control rings (CR), each one enclosing an experimental plot of 2.5 m^2. Each ring consisted of a circular and horizontal plenum made by a corrugated polyethylene pipe, resting on the soil surface, through which CO_2 enriched air was blown on the plot. The target concentration in FR was 550 $\mu mol\ mol^{-1}$. Details on the system are given elsewhere (Miglietta et al., 2001).

Fumigation started in 1998; analyses were performed in the growth seasons 2000 and 2001. Floristic and phenological analyses were performed fortnightly; mowing took place three times per year. Chemical composition of samples was analyzed by Weende and Van Soest methods; digestibility was assessed by the Tilley and Terry method, and the forage energetic value was expressed according to the INRA system, using the conventional "forage units".

Results and discussion

The effects of fumigation can be described as follows:

- CO_2 fumigation enhanced biomass production, with differences among the seasons;
- floristic diversity tended to decrease in FR; in particular, recovery of some species was inhibited after mowing;
- CO_2 fumigation seems to have stimulated the production of perennial species, while this trend was not observed for annual species;
- the mean phenological cycle of the perennial species was very similar in FR and CR; the mean phenological phase of the annual species was more progressed in FR than in CR;
- harvest season strongly influenced all the analyzed parameters; CO_2 fumigation affected protein and fiber content;
- fumigation effects on digestibility varied according to harvest season and plant species; digestibility was more often reduced in Fabaceae, while Poaceae showed contrasting results;
- forage units tend to be reduced in FR.

Conclusions

Although a longer treatment would be necessary to assess long term fumigation effects, yet changes in both species composition and chemical composition are likely to take place; in particular in Fabaceae, elevated CO_2 may result in a poorer quality.

References

Miglietta F. et al., 2001. Environ. Monitoring and Assessment 66:107-127.
Leadley P.W. et al., 1996. Global Change Biology 2:389-397.
Raschi A. et al., 1997. Abstracta Botanica, 21:289-297.

Acknowledgements

The work was in part supported by EU, Contract ENV4-CT97-0503.

A new abatement technique to reduce gaseous and particulate emissions from farm animal house

J. Schulz[1], L. Formosa[1], S. Koch[2], H. Snell[3] & J. Hartung[1*]
[1]*Institute for Animal Hygiene, Animal Welfare and Behaviour of Farm Animals, School of Veterinary Medicine Hanover, Bünteweg 17p, 30559 Hannover, Germany,* [2]*UltraKat AG, Max-Roth-Str. 1, 76571 Gaggenau, Germany,* [3]*Forschungs- und Studienzentrum Weser-Ems der Georg-August-Universität Göttingen, Driverstr. 22, 49377 Vechta, Germany. itt@tiho-hannover.de*

Introduction

It is widely documented that livestock buildings are a source of a wide range of air pollutants which can be both a potential health risk for farm workers and housed animals and harmful to the environment. The most important aerial pollutants are odourants, gases, dust, micro-organisms and endotoxins, also called bioaerosols, which are emitted by way of the exhaust air into the environment, directly polluting the surrounding environment with odours, ammonia (NH_3) and particulates and indirectly contributing to global gaseous inventories (methane,CH_4, nitrous oxide, N_2O).

There exists several techniques capable of cleaning air from aerosols and gaseous pollutants some examples include; air filtration and washing (bio-filters, bio-scrubbers), radiation, ionisation and absorption methods. Although these methods may be effective, they are often too expensive and impractical to merit application in livestock houses.

Materials and methods

This project is investigating the potential benefits of a newly developed abatement technique involving the use of an atmospheric plasma. The breakdown process involves a multitude of complex physical and chemical reactions occurring simultaneously in the plasma phase, the efficiency is partly based on the high electron densities (10^{18} cm^{-3}) within the plasma. An example of a dissociation mechanism is through rapid electron impacts with pollutants (average electron energy 1 to 10 eV). Furthermore, high-energy photons are formed from the discharge (UV, VUV). The high energy photons cause radical formation and subsequent dissociation of molecules. Other resulting products from the air plasma include, the formation of oxidising species such as atomic oxygen, ozone and nitrogen oxides, these substances can modify molecules by oxidation and are known as micro-organism killing agents.

First studies with the plasma generator have involved testing under laboratory conditions and with pig house air. In the laboratory, several manufactured bioaerosols were released into a defined air stream that passed through the plasma phase. The aerosols were captured at the reactor outlet and the living organism content was analysed.

Results and discussion

Preliminary results found bacterial spores were reduced tenfold and 8% of the yeast cells were inactivated. The tests with the pig house air showed the instruments capability in reducing the ammonia content from 25 ppm below the detectable level.

These results show the potential that exists for the air plasma technique as a means of purifying livestock house air from living micro-organisms, gases and odours. However, the investigation is only at the very beginning and so much more research is needed to assess the true capabilities of this method for air purification in the future.

Physiological responses of Holstein and Holstein x Jersey cattle in a grazing system in Argentina

P.E. Leva[1], M.S. García[1], M.A. Veles[1], J. Gandolfo[1] & S.E. Valtorta[2]*
[1]*Facultad de Ciencias Agrarias, Universidad Nacional del Litoral,* [2]*CONICET – INTA, EEA Rafaela Ruta 34 km 227 Rafaela, Santa Fe, Argentina*

Introduction

The objective of the present work were: 1. to assess rectal temperature and respiratory rate difference between morning and afternoon, during the central months of each season in Holstein (H) and 50% Holstein x Jersey (HJ) cows, and 2. to analyze the grazing pattern of H and HJ cows in summer.

Materials and methods

The trial was performed in a dairy farm located in Esperanza, Santa Fe, Argentina (31° 11' south latitude) from April 2002 till January 2003. During the central month of each season 10 H and 10 H J cows were selected. Rectal temperature (RT) and respiration rates (RR) were recorded during am and pm milkings. Differences (afternoon-morning) were analyzed to detect breed effects within each season. During summer, vibracorders were placed on H and HJ cows, to determine the grazing pattern of both groups.

Results and discussion

Table 1 shows RT and RR differences between morning and afternoon in both groups of cows:

Table 1. Rectal temperatures (RT) and respiratory rate (RR) during the experiment.

Breed	Autumn*		Winter*		Spring*		Summer*	
	TR	RR	TR	RR	TR	RR	TR	RR
H	0.65±0.41	8.2±5.02	0.60±0.44	3.0±5.1	1.81±0.58	10.6±7.1	1.51±0.68	30.8±10.5
HJ	0.62±0.43	7.6±6.38	0.42±0.64	4.6±3.4	1.53±0.68	15.3±6.0	1.54±0.69	33.2±10.3

* No statistical differences have been detected

The analysis of summer vibracorders records indicated that both breeds presented peaks at approximately the same time during the day (H: 8 am and 7 pm; HJ: 9 am and 7 pm). However, percentage of activity in H cows was higher in the afternoon (11.67% at 7 pm *vs.* 6.24% at 8 am) as compared to HJ (7.84% at 7 pm vs. 6.98% at 9 am). The pattern for H cows was quite similar to the one that had already been assessed in the same area (Valtorta et al., 1996). Holstein cows presented more activity during the night-time.

Conclusions

No differences in physiological responses or in summer grazing pattern were detected between Holstein and Holstein x Jersey cows.

References

Valtorta, S.E. et al. 1996. Trans. ASAE 39:131-136

Author index

Keyword index

The EAAP Technical Series so far contains the following publications:

- **No. 1. Protein feed for animal production**
  With special reference to Central and Eastern Europe
  edited by C. Février, A. Aumaitre, F. Habe, T. Vares, M. Zjalic
  ISBN 9076998035 – 2001 – 184 pages – € 35 – US$ 39

- **No. 2. Livestock breeding and service organisations**
  With special reference to CEE countries
  edited by J. Boyazoglu, J. Hodges, M. Zjalic, P. Rafai
  ISBN 9076998043 – 2002 – 75 pages – € 25 – US$ 30

- **No. 3. Livestock Farming Systems in Central and Eastern Europe**
  edited by A. Gibon, S. Mihina
  ISBN 9076998299 – 2003 – 264 pages – € 39 – US$ 51

- **No. 4. Image of the Cattle Sector and its Products**
  Role of Breeders Association
  ISBN 9076998337 – 2003 – 80 pages – € 27 – US$ 32

- **No. 5. Foot-and-Mouth Disease: new values, distinct routes**
  edited by A.J. van der Zijpp, M.J.E. Braker, C.H.A.M. Eilers, H. Kieft, S.J. Oosting and T.A. Vogelzang
  ISBN 9076998272 – 2003 – 100 pages – € 30 – US$ 42

- **No. 6. Working animals in agriculture and transport**
  A collection of some current research and development observations
  edited by R.A. Pearson, P. Lhoste, M. Saastamoinen, W. Martin-Rosset
  ISBN 9076998256 – 2003 – 208 pages – € 40 – US$ 53

- **No. 7. Interactions between climate and animal production**
  edited by N. Lacetera, U. Bernabucci, H.H. Khalifa, B. Ronchi and A. Nardone
  ISBN 9076998264 – 2003 – 128 pages – € 35 – US$ 39

These publications are available at:
Wageningen Academic Publishers
P.O. Box 220
6700 AE Wageningen
The Netherlands

sales@WageningenAcademic.com
www.WageningenAcademic.com

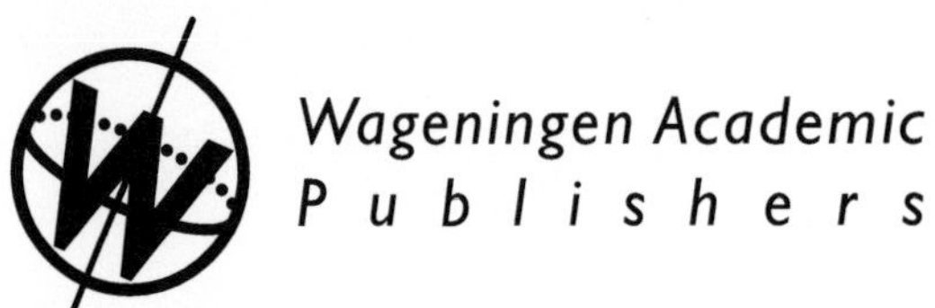

Printed in the United States
by Baker & Taylor Publisher Services